Doctors
Triumphs, Trials and Tragedies

Dr John Wright

JoJo
PUBLISHING

Doctors: Triumphs, Trials and Tragedies
Dr. John Wright

Published by JoJo Publishing
First published 2012

'Yarra's Edge'
2203/80 Lorimer Street
Docklands VIC 3008
Australia

JoJo
🖋
PUBLISHING

Email: jo-media@bigpond.net.au or visit www.jojopublishing.com

© Dr. John Wright

JoJo Publishing

Editor: Ormé Harris
Designer / typesetter: Chameleon Print Design

Printed in Singapore by KHL Printing

National Library of Australia Cataloguing-in-Publication data

Author:	Wright, John S. (John Saxon)
Title:	Doctors : triumphs, trials and tragedies / John Wright.
Edition:	1st ed.
ISBN:	9780980871098 (pbk.)
Subjects:	Physicians--Malpractice--Case studies.
	Medical personnel--Malpractice--Case studies.
Dewey Number:	344.0411

About the Author

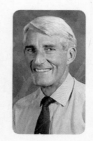

John Wright graduated with high medical honours from the University of Sydney in 1955. He was awarded Fellowship of the Royal Australasian College of Surgeons in 1959. He spent six years at the Royal Prince Alfred Hospital where he was surgical tutor to three students' colleges, senior surgical registrar and surgical superintendent before departing for overseas studies of chest and heart surgery in England and the USA.

He was appointed senior cardiothoracic surgical registrar in the Liverpool region of England and later took up cardiac surgical Fellowships of the distinguished universities at Stanford, California and Ann Arbor, Michigan.

His special cardiothoracic interest was open-heart surgery, particularly for the correction of childhood defects.

As an Australian with unique awards of Fellowships of the American Colleges of Surgeons, the American College of Chest Physicians and Senior Membership of the American Society of Thoracic Surgeons, he was invited to a specialist cardiothoracic surgical post at the Teaching Hospitals of the University of New South Wales in Sydney in the early 1960s. He was appointed to the first Australian professorial post in cardiothoracic surgery in 1969. He headed his department, tutored and examined all student levels, wrote two textbooks and more than 200 peer-reviewed articles on children's heart surgery and consulted at nine major Sydney hospitals.

In 1985, he was invited to fill the Foundation Chair of Paediatric Cardiac Surgery at the Prince of Wales (Sydney) Children's Hospital. After establishing that department, he rejected further public hospital appointments and took up senior consulting posts in Sydney, Brisbane, Canberra and Darwin. He is the author of three textbooks.

Preamble

Material in this book has been on the public record for many years without known challenge. The great majority of 'case histories' are transcriptions of that information and rely on reports of the NSW Medical Board and its tribunals, court documents, judgements, biographies, letters and reputable media reports. The bibliography lists those sources.

The first Australian case history (Chapter 10), headed George Davidson, John Beveridge, Matthew Crawford and the Prince of Wales Hospital concerns an entirely different type of medical conduct (sham peer review). Its inclusion here invites the reader to consider the moral ambiguities of such procedures. All affected doctors have been given the benefit of the doubt where irrefutable evidence is not available. Even then, selection of case material has been based only on features of unusual interest. Doctors' detailed defences against criticism are unknown. Those who have been investigated by statutory authorities for incidents in their practices tend to have, overall, unblemished records of service. Every one of them has had experience of academic and clinical triumphs.

Details of current professional status of each doctor are unknown to the author. His assessment of them is unbiased by the specific incidents detailed here to the extent that none is unconditionally and necessarily evidence of an irreversible major, systemic flaw of character. It has been accepted that each one has earned respect for most or all of his or her professional life.

The case histories have been presented objectively without presumption, personal opinion, or moral judgement or implied criticism by the author. Here again, none represents an endorsement of opinions published elsewhere in the media or in disciplinary reports. If unfairness or inaccuracy is perceived, the author will be glad to review the relevant text.

Essentially, I am reporting information which has been available elsewhere for years without published objection. I am not privy to additional material and I am not bound to accept that information, whatever its source. I am therefore acting as a reporter of what happened to those named and I have not questioned any party about his or her experiences. Hence, I have no additional facts to disclose and I cannot verify, accept or deny what was decided by those who investigated events and formed opinions based on them. In one case of sham peer review, the information has been freely available for 25 years and was widely and repeatedly published by the victim 14 years ago with no later objection by those involved in the 'review'.

Table of Contents

Preface

The great majority of doctors are essentially honourable, generous, reliable and effective. Many of them work in sheltered environments such as laboratories where they are never likely to encounter temptations to misbehave professionally and scarcely understand how others might feel and act differently. All of them have been high achievers, prepared to wait 10 or 20 years after secondary schooling before being able to command a reasonable income. Regardless of that, there is a perception that many of them are wealthy, off-hand, politically powerful and snobbish. In fact, regardless of the media's and lawyers' preoccupation with doctors' negligence and other sins, they are still trusted and respected much more widely than any other professional group.

Doctors are unique in what they know and can do and people admire and envy them for it but that is no different from how they admire airline pilots or nurses or dental surgeons or nuclear physicists or many other human pursuits. One large difference is that doctors are highly privileged — they are almost intuitively believed to be trustworthy, honest, reliable healers of the sick and, above all, concerned. But there is another unique difference. If necessary and done appropriately, they are required and allowed to 'touch' patients intimately, both physically and psychologically. In fact, the skill of physically touching a frightened, sick person for the purpose of diagnosis and treatment divides doctors generally in a fundamental fashion. Some of them are never comfortable or comforting in that respect. Hence there is a natural and chosen primary separation into groups and specialties according to that capability.

1

Almost all of them began their medical studies with an ambition and expectation to make the world somehow a better place. Are the risk-takers amongst them any different from those in other jobs who cross a boundary into the dangerous territory of being investigated, penalised and, perhaps, sent into professional oblivion? Of course, their possible foibles are not generically different from any other human's weaknesses. Greed, dishonesty, lust and lack of scruple in doctors are no different from others but flaws are possibly more at odds with their general behaviour, original incentives, aspirations and belief systems.

No doubt their privileges offer different and more accessible opportunities to stray from safe paths than others might — more tempting because liberties may be more personal and trust is assumed to be part of what they represent and who they are. Unlike many other employments, the practice of medicine generally has an earlier end-point than, say, law but similar to that of an airline pilot. Something worthwhile and rewarding is hoped for before the shelf-life of serviceability is near or reached.

Perhaps time runs out too soon and there is nowhere else to go that quite fills the gap between medicine, which can be so exotic, admirable and noteworthy, and the hum-drum of retirement or a menial part-time practice with less overt and available psychological rewards. Perhaps, too, there is a sense of enforced haste and an unrecognised inducement to stretch limits. The characteristics of this behaviour and its penalties are examined here. The issue of 'group' malfeasance by cabals is touched on as the final tragic distortion of noble hopes in all concerned.

Chapter 1

How the medical game is played

There were 60,000 doctors registered in Australia in 2007, most of them working in major cities in New South Wales or Victoria. Of the 30,000 in New South Wales, 40% were in general practice and another 40% were in specialist practice or in training for it. During that year, about 3,500 new registrations were listed, including 200 overseas-trained doctors.

On the other side of the equation, 2,250 doctors' names were removed from the NSW register voluntarily or by death. There was, therefore, a net gain of about 1,250 registered doctors in NSW.

Complaints

In general terms, medical 'misconduct' concerns 'negligence' or 'gross negligence', depending on features such as wilful or wanton acts, recklessness, failure to give proper care as expected by peers or to practise diligent supervision. These issues are considered in most 'malpractice' claims against doctors, nurses and other health professionals. The State of New York lists 50 such possible behaviours in its doctors. The number and severity of default are taken into account in grading offences. 'Malpractice' usually implies that an injury has followed 'misconduct'.

'Incompetence' refers to a lack of necessary knowledge or ability in care and often requires repetition to invoke significant penalties. On the other hand, 'impairment' emphasises that a 'disability' is inadequately managed by a doctor. It may be physical, requiring selected medical employment, or result from self-induced limitation, such as substance abuse, without adequate monitoring or rehabilitation.

'Sexual abuse' is regarded as a 'moral' limitation which results from any improper physical contact between a doctor and a patient, or suggestive behaviour and words inviting sexual acts. Less egregious misconduct includes fraud, civil crimes, inappropriate advertising and the abandonment of a patient without adequate explanation and alternative carer arrangements existing.

Every year, roughly one thousand of the 30,000 doctors registered in NSW have a complaint about them referred to the Medical Board. Half of the complaints are thought to need no disciplinary action. Of the remainder, 50% are investigated and a penalty is imposed, ranging from a reprimand up to deregistration for the worst offences. Of all the complaints made, deregistration follows in about one percent.

Most primary complaints are for misconduct such as fraud, sexual and drug offences, improper prescribing, physical and/or mental impairment and generally unsatisfactory performance. Colleagues and employers contribute some of them but the great majority of complaints come from patients. A few seem frivolous or malicious.

Some of the most difficult cases are deemed emergencies requiring special powers for the *protection of public health and safety*. In its terminology about those, medical boards commonly refer to *'unethical, reckless, wilful or criminal behaviour ... in clinical and non-clinical senses'*.

In 2005, the *Sydney Morning Herald* reported that one in every three Australian anaesthetists has a significant mishap each year — three times the number recorded against any other medical group. Of those, one in five led to litigation or financial settlement. Elsewhere in this book is further comment on difficulties with anaesthesia in hospital practice.

In clear cases of fabrication of credentials, opinions hold that such misrepresentation deserves immediate censure and possibly dismissal.

Foreign graduates

With the vast publicity directed at the conduct of foreign graduates in Australia, particularly in the state of Queensland where the names of Patel, Haneef, Popov and others have attracted headlines, it is no surprise that the Australian Doctors Trained Overseas Association has expressed fears that its members may be stigmatised for being foreign. Those fears have been exacerbated by the conviction of Jayant Patel for manslaughter and grievous bodily harm during his surgical career in Queensland.

In English-speaking countries, particularly, there is a vigorous industry of medical recruitment agencies finding foreign doctors to fill medical vacancies. Most of the agents have little real knowledge of health systems. They seek expressions of interest, in Australia and New Zealand alone, from thousands of overseas-trained doctors who apply for work-permits and jobs. Of these, at least 200 become registered at some level, albeit temporarily.

From more than 150 of these recruitment agencies, hundreds of medical credentials are passed on to potential employers without exhaustive checking of applicants' experience, medical degrees or history. Proper investigation at any level of Queensland health administration would have immediately revealed that [Dr] Jayant Patel had been twice banned in the US before he applied for and was appointed to a senior surgical position at the Bundaberg Base Hospital. Similar concealment is not too uncommon in job applications from Australian doctors to work in Australia, generally because there is no established authority, apart from employing hospitals, which wishes to scrupulously investigate such vital issues when staff shortages are large and endemic.

The Sunday Times (David Rose) of January 23, 2007 reported that rogue doctors and thousands of other health professionals who have been struck off registers for misconduct in other European countries are able to work in Britain because there is no mechanism to warn employers of their histories. A certificate of good standing and evidence of recognised medical training suffice to work in Britain. Although a minority exploit free-movement rights and put patients at risk, the system is inadequate to cull out those unfit to practise for any reason or lacking language skills or with past records of professional misconduct or even criminality.

Similarly, the London *Daily Mail* of March 29, 2009 reported that Ireland had become a 'safe haven for rogue doctors' who had been deregistered in the UK; remarkably, the Irish Medical Council cannot deregister such doctors without an enquiry of its own, though aware of them from UK records. Clearly, a common registration procedure is urgently overdue for geographically related regions. The Australian Medical Board (AHPRA) came into operation on July 1, 2010 partly in an effort to minimise concealment of registration issues by movement of doctors between states and territories.

Similar reservations about screening systems have been expressed by Scottish authorities who have discovered that one doctor had been accessing, with no known purpose or authority, the electronic records of prominent people.

It implies no discrimination to observe that doctors whose names are not of Anglo-Saxon origin are disproportionately likely to be the subject of complaints. Whether that relates to less effective medical education, communication defects, discrimination or different cultural, qualifying and practice behaviour is not clear.

Legal trawling and information services in Australia

There are vast numbers of legal machines dedicated constantly, completely and specifically to the discovery of any blemish at any time on the record of any doctor. These machines offer 'obligation-free' legal advice to patients in an attempt to convert them to claimants. They specialise in *medical negligence — how to make an official complaint and how to access health and case-law expertise.*

Just as ambulance-chasers offer a quick and easy avenue to getting information and justice for injured persons, legal information services publish spectacular details of medical disciplinary actions and the nature of doctors' misconduct — information collected primarily from the media. They promise to provide their tempted clients with extensive information in any type of medical misadventure or error and, particularly, in how to go about making a claim for compensation: *just complete the contact form and a solicitor will be in touch with you.*

That magnetic invitation reassures claimants of their need for and the easy and possibly free availability of a full range of lawyers who know the key concerns: '*Make no mistake: medical errors can be deadly serious; anonymity and transparency in reporting medical error; the role of information in reducing and penalising medical error*'. Those offers encourage in sick or injured people the notions of cash, revenge against wayward doctors and others and even a crusade to 'clean up' the medical profession. It is of interest that, after years of conjecture, evidence now suggests that so-called PTSD (post-traumatic stress disorder) after major injury rarely improves until a culprit is established and compensation paid.

The dragnet on offer takes further pains to remind patients of the various parts of their body which might be damaged by medical intervention. Paediatric and obstetric matters get special mention. In their advertising material, these sources stress three powerful themes: firstly, the sorts of *complaints* to make about health delivery; secondly, the sorts of medical *mistakes* that might occur; thirdly, the amount of *damages* that have been awarded elsewhere as precedents. All are reference points for calculating the nature and size of possible claims. Some published examples are presented in the following ways:

Snippets of triggering material derived from typical media headlines

- *More than 2200 medication errors (in) South Australia's major hospitals in the past year (2007).*
- *Avoidable hospital catastrophes killed 38 Victorians in the past year.*
- *... non-fatal cases included swabs and instruments left inside patients, giving wrong blood, surgery performed on incorrect body part, medication mix-ups, flawed procedures, poor communication, human error.*
- *500 mistakes were reported at the Royal North Shore Hospital leading to serious injury or death.*
- *36 patient deaths from negligence or catastrophic failures in the medical system.*
- *[In 759 public hospitals Australia-wide in 2004-05] there were 'missing records, ambiguous or illegible documentation, inadequate training, problems with faulty rules, policies and procedures.' [It was emphasised that information was not confined to public hospitals.]*
- *130 needless patient deaths in 2004-2005 classed as 'blunders in hospitals' shame-file'.*
- *'... hospital bungles ... killing scores'.*
- *[In Western Australia, lack of transparency in the reporting of patient death or damage:] '42 hospital patients died or were left with permanent disabilities in the past financial year as a result of clinical errors'.*
- *[In New South Wales:] '... up to 130,000 patients are being harmed or experience near-misses each year. There are an estimated 8,000 deaths each year as a result of medical errors, (five times) more than the annual road toll ...'*
- *The Royal Melbourne Hospital recorded 1,217 medication errors in 2005-2006.*

Professor Merrilyn Walton, who once headed the New South Wales Health Care Complaints Commission, though not a doctor, was quoted as saying: *System errors* [mean that] *governments are going to have to be brave and deal with this violation of basic standards of care.* The NSW Clinical Excellence Commission [CEC] found that defects in *policies and procedures* in hospitals were to blame for a quarter of all notifications to it. Oddly enough, in all health systems, falls were the commonest single type of incident reported, usually occurring in already-disabled patients. To what extent they represent a management problem is by no means clear when staffing numbers are almost universally insufficient.

Whom to pursue and for how much?

This category of information includes examples of the sorts of doctors and events that patients should be on the look-out for in media headlines. Again, these factors give clues as to what range of compensation is possible. There is no aspect of 'doctor-failure' that cannot be investigated and possibly exploited to the financial advantage of patients and/or to their grieving families and their lawyers.

Such opportunistic advice does not necessarily relate to a doctor's personal shortcomings in issues such as 'misconduct', 'performance', 'safety' or 'ethics'. Those aspects tend to be the province of disciplinary and regulatory medical bodies. 'Pain and loss' seem much easier to tolerate when a 'fault' can be found to warrant compensation.

Australian Legal Information — Health and Medical Law, 2006-2007, referring to Australian incidents which were *directly or indirectly* related to doctors' [and other health workers'] actions or lack thereof, included the following quotes which were clearly intended to fuel resentment, alarm and revenge-seeking by patients. The majority of these references offered an easily-identified target for attack:

- *Three Queensland doctors face disciplinary action and possible deregistration after … unsatisfactory professional conduct (which) contributed to the death of a mother of four.*
- *Queensland's former Chief Health Officer … faces disciplinary action for his role in the Dr Jayant Patel scandal at Bundaberg …*
- *Complaints over nurses increased in Victoria by almost 20% in the past year. There were 162 complaints and 24 nurses were suspended. Misappropriation of medications doubled between 2005 and 2006.*
- *A foreign medical graduate was deregistered for at least ten years for 'failed abortion, ruptured uteruses, a botched circumcision, poor post-operative care and incorrect cancer diagnosis'.*
- *The Victorian Government investigates how its medical board approved an overseas-trained doctor who was later found to be 'unsuitable' to work at two regional hospitals.*
- *A junior doctor in Victoria administered an overdose of glucose to a baby, leaving the child brain damaged. A lack of knowledge and competence were detected and criticised but the doctor was not deregistered [due to her inexperience].*
- *A psychiatrist paid a former patient $100,000 to conceal a seven-year sexual affair. He was banned from practising for at least two years for a 'breach of trust, misuse of power and exploitation of a former patient's vulnerability'.*
- *A senior Queensland doctor responded too slowly to an emergency, which contributed to a patient's death. He was 'too far away from the hospital for a timely response to gravely ill patients while on call'.*
- *A pathologist misreported specimens on hundreds of patients at Tamworth and Wollongong Hospitals. The investigation required the audit of 7,432 pathology tests performed between 1991 and 2001. Although there were unnecessary operations performed and delays in the start of treatment as a result of his reports, there was difficulty in drawing any definite connection*

between the mistaken pathology reports and any patient death. The pathologist was banned from practising as a pathologist in New South Wales.

- A conference on safety and quality in health care heard that random drug tests had been recommended by a US expert to detect doctors' substance abuse.
- A North Adelaide doctor demonstrated 'serious disregard for the well-being of his patients' by his reluctance to transfer medical notes to another doctor and by advertising that he could help patients win compensation cases by referring them to lawyers who would maximise their claims. Also, his letterhead indicated membership of professional organisations to which he did not belong and he issued inappropriate medical certificates.
- A trainee neurosurgeon was convicted of child pornography charges, sentenced to five months (suspended) jail and was dismissed from a neurosurgical training program. That prevented him from practising surgery in Australia again. He was not regarded as a paedophile. Stress and anxiety were considered significant causative factors. He was ordered regular psychiatric treatment for at least ten years and was banned from treating children for the same period.
- All South Australian doctors are now forbidden to accept gifts, to form sexual or personal relationships with patients or to pressure them to take up private health insurance.
- A Queensland orthopaedic surgeon was discovered to have served six months in a US jail in 1982 for raping a nurse. He failed to reveal the conviction to the Queensland health authorities in an application for registration. The Health Minister recommended that a criminal history check be conducted on all 14,000 doctors working in Queensland.
- A former Queensland health chief sought taxpayer-funded cover for his legal costs in a medical board investigation of his failure to detect Dr Jayant Patel's past US record of deregistration.

- *A child psychiatrist used a bizarre form of electric shock therapy to punish young children. He promised never to practise again.*
- *An Adelaide forensic pathologist wrongly blamed a car accident for the deaths of a couple who were later found to have been murdered.*
- *A Campbelltown Hospital patient had a healthy breast removed instead of the opposite breast which contained cancer.*

Prevention of indiscriminate litigation

These instances of misconduct and misadventure are alarming and seemingly endless although their real frequency is relatively small as we shall see later. Disciplinary bodies and 'doctor-watchers' of all sorts expect, very reasonably, that their policies and interventions will act as deterrents to would-be offenders. But to make matters worse, it is commonly claimed that medical errors are concealed or under-reported by observers as a result of the deceptive 'culture of medicine' rather than from a fear of malpractice claims. How that can be confirmed is impossible to know but the media and lawyers are prone to that presumption.

It has often been suggested without any real evidence that more 'classical' student teaching is a key to reducing medical misconduct and to promoting 'transparency' about errors. Senior doctors may look back in anger on medical school teaching of basic anatomy, for example, being cut by 80% in recent years to make way for 'touchy-feely' topics such as cultural sensitivity, community medicine and communication. That comment does not suggest that the teaching of those is not important but a more practical balance of curriculums might produce more objective and 'impersonal' doctors. After all, post-mortem human dissection is usually the first professional contact a student has with another human's body parts but, remarkably, many anatomy departments in major universities have no human anatomists on staff.

One large doctors' group has made a submission to the Federal Government listing arguments from more than two dozen professors, consultants and medical academics for a rethink on medical education. They fear that highly 'socialised' interactions between teachers and students [first-name terms, no white coats, open sharing of personal experiences, gifting, quasi-psychotherapy and unchaperoned examinations] might more easily create an environment where improper and potentially dangerous values and relationships may originate and flourish. Interestingly, it has lately been postulated that poor student performance might have a correlation with misconduct after graduation.

Comparing hospital and general practice

General practitioners are more liable to complaints than any other doctors. Dr Meredith Makeham reported in the Medical Journal of Australia that a mistake occurs in one of every 1,000 visits to a GP. This may represent under-reporting when some errors are never admitted because no harm arises from them. A lack of disclosure in such cases might be rationalised, at least by unlucky doctors, simply because of the insignificance of the errors, their 'freak' causation and a wish to avoid alarming a patient unnecessarily.

Unfortunately for its practitioners, medical practice is an inherently risky activity and there are some factors which affect all doctors to some extent in the conduct of their medical practices. One half of all adverse events occurring in hospitals, and a larger proportion of those arising in general practice, are probably avoidable by changes in practice management, billing procedures and staff communication but none of those measures excuses frank misconduct.

Regardless of the enormous number of complaints made about medical care, few of the untoward events occurring in public hospitals are deemed 'serious' or have a mortal outcome.

How these events affect a doctor's life can only be assessed by examining the bio-ethics of medical practice — how they have developed over the centuries, the accepted principles of safe management competing with constant opportunities to exploit patients and situations, the occurrence of coincidental, unavoidable and harmful events and their constant scrutiny by governing bodies and lawyers to find exploitable flaws.

Extremes of doctor blaming

On 29 February 2008, Robert Kaplan, a Wollongong 'forensic psychiatrist', wrote a synopsis for the *Sydney Morning Herald* of his intended publication in October 2008: *'Medical murder: the disturbing phenomenon of doctors who kill'*. The harshly pejorative title was unlikely to encourage acceptance of any *new social contract* [his term] between doctors and patients. Indeed, he recognises that *self-interested agents, regulatory and legal ... urge patients to complain, sue and seek redress.* If his intention is to change this culture, the evidence for that is ominously otherwise, particularly in regard to his unmitigated denunciation of (then Dr) Jayant Patel who was judged guilty of serious offences in 2010 and penalised in Queensland.

An exhaustive and truly peer-tested evaluation of all conditions of this surgeon's surgical service, and of his responses to criticisms, was not then available. He was in a US gaol for months while awaiting extradition to the jurisdiction of Australian Federal authorities. Inevitably, he sought full access to case-notes and particulars of claims against him. Some of his critics were apparently less than enthusiastic about providing them for undisclosed reasons so that the extradition process was protracted.

In the context of social contracts, the targeting of medicine as an area for blame suggests a unique paradox compounded of history, religion, the evolution of bioethics, the uniquely personal character of medical practice and an abiding belief that good medical care is a birthright. It is impossible to believe that an airline pilot, a politician, a government, a bureaucrat, a mariner, an arsonist, a corporation, an extremist, a motor driver, a physician or a psychiatrist who might wreak just as much enduring physical, social, emotional and financial injury to individuals and society as is claimed against Jayant Patel would ever attract such destructive, incompletely-sourced and indelible judgements as Patel endured before his trial began.

It was expected that Dr Kaplan's published story, unlike its menacing, dark title, would throw light into places where profound prejudgements persisted for no obvious reason. In laymen's terms, therefore, while Patel's detailed defences were then unknown, haste to condemn him completely and unconditionally might well have been tempered.

Difficult dividing lines

As Jayant Patel's manslaughter conviction shows, medical mistakes are increasingly regarded as 'criminal' acts, which must reflect society's hardening expectations of doctors' performance. An editorial in the *British Medical Journal* has asked: 'Does the punishment [adequately] fit the crime?' Indeed, recent investigations into the deaths of prisoners-of-war in Iraq, for example, have revealed such serious human rights issues as to encourage a belief in criminality in medical conduct. Evaluation of cases in which prisoners may have died from mistreatment or under suspicious but concealed circumstances suggests there was some collusion between the military and supposedly impartial doctors.

Investigations will entail consideration of what constitutes 'legitimate' medical [and military] purpose in regard to techniques of interrogation of prisoners, whatever that term may mean to an individual doctor. Ultimately, of course, decisions to assist or resist improper forms of interrogation should be the personal choice of doctors and others who are involved in such provocative situations.

Elsewhere, there has been much distressing information arising from New Orleans where, in the wake of Cyclone Katrina, marauding criminals were heavily armed from looted gun-stores while medical staff were confronted by terminally ill patients who had nowhere to go to escape certain destruction. It has been freely admitted by doctors who were caught up in this drama that they judged it their humane duty [asking for the mercy of God rather than their peers] to resort to a benign but urgent form of euthanasia. They saw no other way to spare unsalvageable, menaced patients the almost certain inevitability of a horrifying death by gunshot, rape or drowning.

There is nothing new in that challenge, perhaps, but Katrina focused world attention on the everlasting dilemmas that plague doctors, especially those working in wars and civilian areas of supreme hazard. The rules of conduct learned in medical schools and early practice cannot always determine proper responses as easily as a tribunal might in the cold light of reasonable argument and the compassionate paradigms of 'normal' society. Nor may those rules apply comfortably to modern society's recurring disasters, many of which carry sudden, extreme and novel dimensions of challenge to medical personnel.

Jack Kevorkian graduated from the University of Michigan Medical School in 1952. In the 1980s he wrote articles on the ethics of euthanasia. In 1987 he advertised in Detroit newspapers as a physician-consultant for 'death counselling'. Between 1990 and 1998, he possibly assisted in the deaths of about 100 terminally-ill people and, for that, became known as the *'Doctor of Death'*. The patients allegedly killed themselves by pressing a button which released drugs or chemicals into a vein or into their lungs.

Kevorkian was deregistered in Michigan in 1991 and was tried many times for assisting suicide. On November 23, 1998, he showed, on national television, a film depicting the voluntary euthanasia of a man with an irreversible, debilitating disease.

While not licensed to practise medicine at the time, but with consent from the patient, Kevorkian was seen administering a lethal injection. He was charged with murder and improper possession of a controlled substance. He was sentenced to 10-25 years in prison but was released eight years later. He has never been re-registered.

[To be more precise, Kevorkian's pejorative nickname (*Doctor of Death*) described his chosen *'specialty'* — quite a different matter from the *'Dr Death'* title accorded to Jayant Patel by the media and others for his alleged sins long before evidence was given to a court. Elsewhere in Australia, there is a *'Butcher of Bega'* awaiting enquiry and legal judgement in 2010 — again a maximally emotive label that sells media products profusely.]

In early 2011, a major innovation occurred in the 'ethical' conduct of global war in its broadest context. In Libya, Colonel Gaddafi's personal survival was overtly threatened by US and NATO military intervention in a rebellion. At the same time, Osama bin Laden was summarily executed by US forces in Pakistan and his body buried at sea. It seems that the rules of war are suddenly changing in momentous ways.

Chapter 2

Guardians of souls and bodies

Ancient times

When and why the concept of medical ethics began is unknown but it was accepted in the Muslim world of the 9th and 10th centuries AD that physicians had obligations towards their patients, whatever their wealth or social situation. One authority described doctors as *guardians of souls and bodies* and emphasised the importance of general conduct, the value of so-called remedies, the dignity of the profession at large and the need for proper qualifications. Attention was concentrated on the need for *removal of corruption among physicians.*

A century later, al-Razi introduced many practical medical and psychological concepts. He vigorously attacked charlatans and fake doctors who roamed the countryside selling potions. He had little respect for the highly educated doctors who pretended to have power to cure all sicknesses and insisted on a form of 'continuing medical education' for physicians. He excused those who failed to cure cancer and leprosy and summarised his views like this: *The doctor's aim is to do good, even to our enemies, so much more to our friends, and my profession forbids us to do harm to our kindred, as it is instituted for the benefit and welfare of the human race, and God imposed on physicians the oath not to compose mortiferous remedies.*

There was about one physician for every 300 inhabitants of Baghdad in 931AD, many of them enjoying the patronage of rulers. Above all else, the training of a good doctor meant developing proper behaviour. Inept, fraudulent physicians and quacks invited the development of rules to control their practices. Connection with a hospital was a mark of eminence. By the 12th century AD, many self-taught physicians were working in teaching hospitals in Baghdad, Damascus and Cairo and were claiming priorities in knowledge and patient care.

Inevitably, the curriculums and training of physicians were not standardised at that time. There were certainly inspectors of public services and chief physicians whose credentials and specific duties are unknown but they were concerned with civic matters such as street cleaning and maintaining healthy water supplies.

During the reign of Saladin, a physician in Aleppo wrote of the need for supervision of the medical community. He insisted that physicians should take the Hippocratic Oath and accept its authority. Centuries earlier, bone and eye doctors were required to fully comprehend a textbook written by Galen before they were considered educated. It was perhaps the beginning of an acceptance that a physician in the medieval, Islamic world was granted a licence only by following some sort of defined medical curriculum.

On the contrary, in Europe there was little or no evidence of ethical, medical concepts during the difficult and protracted evolution of medical thinking and standards of the Middle Ages. Even so, it seems that both Eastern and Western medical worlds were equally aware of the Hippocratic Oath and its implications regardless of how well they were observed during the centuries before the Royal College of Surgeons of England was founded in 1800.

Refining the art
Broadly speaking, medical ethics today is the study of moral values as they apply to doctors and other health workers.

Inevitably, ethics relate to the history of medicine as well as to philosophy, theology and sociology. Jewish, Christian and Muslim physicians of the 12th century embraced some Hippocratic principles long before they understood why they had similar principles. In the 18th and 19th centuries, Europeans became more conscious of codes of conduct and medical jurisprudence from the publications of Dr Thomas Percival in England. The American Medical Association adopted its first code of ethics in 1847, 15 years before the American Civil War.

Of course, the values of Hippocrates do not provide answers to many questions which confront a practising doctor in the 21st century but they provide a framework for understanding how to treat others. After all, history has shown repeatedly that there may be no satisfactory solution to many dilemmas in medical science and, as with all professional groups, conflicts will inevitably occur between doctors and their patients' families, lawyers, governors and their consciences.

The powerful concept of *informed consent* has become ever more complicated by the ambition to harvest organs and tissues from consenting, very recently dead or already brain-dead humans for grafting into those who cannot survive without new organs. Ideally, consent is personal or surrogate. Powers of Attorney and Living Wills are part of the way through the mass of potential difficulties in such matters and involved doctors need to be seen to have observed every possible scruple. Transplant history has certainly showed disturbing irregularities when expediency and haste have overtaken good sense and principle.

Confidentiality, even in testimony under oath, is a principle usually applied to the content of communications between doctors and their patients. Patient privacy extends to complex situations issues such as revealing the existence of a sexually transmitted disease in a patient who refuses to reveal the diagnosis to a partner, or in discussing the termination of pregnancy in an under-aged patient without the knowledge of her parents. In trying to preserve

21

an over-arching medical concept of 'doing good to humanity', these tricky circumstances inevitably pose profound dilemmas that often defy satisfying resolution.

A crucial proposition in Hippocrates' oath, which most Western medical graduates take at the time of their licensing, is: *first, do no harm'*. The simplicity of that phrase belies the great difficulties that arise in specific value judgements. There are many stark 'conduct' issues which plague every doctor who treats patients. The management of grossly incapacitated patients in New Orleans, for example, presented the ultimate challenge to doctors who practised a form of euthanasia to spare bed-ridden patients new agonies.

A common 'humanity' issue arises in clinical practice when a patient who is certain to die early and has pain and suffering of the worst kind, may require doses of narcotics which, undoubtedly and knowingly, will hasten death while also affording the only possible humanity. No doubt, such matters challenge any jurisdiction and much reliance has to be placed on the quantity and quality of communication between a doctor and other parties concerned, including other medical practitioners.

Those who would presume to become involved in advising on and deciding such delicate issues may find themselves on committees composed of doctors and other medical professionals, clergy, ethicists, philosophers, lawyers and administrators — all trying to 'adjudicate' on matters of profound ethical conflict. Many of them have little or no personal experience of the issues about which they must form opinions but their decisions need to take account of cultural and spiritual differences between individuals. Ultimately, they must be, personally and in conscience, invulnerable to criticism because of their own past misadventures. They also need to have no bias or conflict of interest in making judgements and to have a substantial parity with other practitioners in professional and related life experiences.

Chapter 3

Hippocrates in the 21st century

S ome of the issues raised in this chapter might seem remote from the day-to-day experience of most doctors but, sooner or later, any of them might become involved in issues of life and death when the path of proper conduct requires deep understanding and guidance.

'Simple' Payola

The burgeoning industry of 'kick-backs' occurring between doctors and pharmaceutical companies threatens to involve a huge range of medical practitioners who might have overlooked that industries which manufacture and supply medications and tools hope to be rewarded by a doctor's recommendation and use of their products.

The Australian newspaper of July 10, 2010 reported that a 'middle-man' company, creating 'an illusion of independence', organised 'training programs' for doctors which significantly boosted sales of Pfizer Australia products. The statement was removed from the 'private company's' website a month later when questions were raised about the 'probity of drug company-sponsored medical education and the prescribing habits of doctors'.

It was also reported that in a 15 month period, big pharmaceutical companies had spent $75 million in Australia on doctors' education. It was further stated that 12,000 GPs had undertaken a 'mental health program' of which Pfizer became a 'commercial partner' in 2001 while a major Sydney University research institute, headed by a prominent doctor who had helped establish such programs, had an 'ongoing commercial relationship' in the program.

In the United States, between 10 and 20 billion dollars are spent annually on drug marketing alone. Doctors might also be rewarded for referring their patients for medical tests more often than a practitioner who has no such 'contract' with diagnostic laboratories. To further complicate matters, more subtle inducements may include gifts, food and drink, medical education costs, conference fees, drug samples and sexual opportunities.

Kick-backs and their variants apply no less to doctors than to others involved in commercial dealing. Conferences fill great halls with state-of-the-art exhibitions manned by attractive and obliging sales people offering information by day and relaxing company at the cocktail hour. Doctors can attend lectures sponsored by companies which manufacture the materials they use and, later, provide homely interviews in their surgeries with attractive people to educate them in their prescribing habits.

Fifty percent of the 'continuing medical education' of GPs in Britain is said to be funded by drug companies. US drug companies invest a billion dollars a year in doctors' 'education'. In Australia, costs are possibly counted in millions of dollars a year. Whether or not this is the best way for doctors to learn about new drugs and equipment is doubtful but it is a very pleasant, quick method of trying. Benefits of one drug company's product over another are rarely obvious in daily use but a glossy brochure and a few free packs of tablets certainly refresh the prescribing memories of busy doctors.

The staging of conferences by pharmaceutical companies with speakers to deliver educational material is not always a simple ethical matter either. It could suggest a benign brain-washing of doctors by biased presentations, even though conference organisers and drug companies insist that all their nominated speakers are asked to be entirely impartial.

An academic variation on payola

In 2009, the US Government sued 20 cardiologists for their involvement in a kick-back scheme where they were given professorial titles and salaries by a university ostensibly for working in teaching, research and patient-care. It seems that the cardiologists were really being paid for directing their patients to the university hospital in order to increase its patient numbers. This is a contravention of the rules of referral of Medicare patients to a hospital. Reparations have been offered by the doctors but many details of their rewards have yet to be examined.

Preferred devices

Australian authorities are investigating donations made by US companies to surgeons and major hospitals in Melbourne [and elsewhere] to encourage the exclusive use of their products, such as artificial hips and knees and spinal implants. Clearly, these probably create a serious conflict of interest. A senior doctor in Melbourne estimated that: *contracts that are given for exclusive* [supply] *of surgical articles, without their being tendered for in public hospitals … are worth hundreds of thousands* [of dollars yearly]. It has also been claimed that threats had been levelled at hospital staff who refused to employ products of one company only.

The US government has found that five of the biggest medical implant companies paid $222 million dollars to doctors in 2007 to get their products used exclusively. Some surgeons received as much as $1 million from a single company. Guilty companies have now agreed to pay $310 million in fines and have promised to tell patients of any links that they have to medical instrument companies. Likewise, the companies are required to declare annually how much they have given individual doctors in cash or equivalents. It is difficult to think of a drug which could not become preferred by a doctor after adequate inducements from its manufacturer — assuming that it is not dangerous, is similarly priced, as effective as and no more prone to complications than any similar drug.

In 2009, the Australian Orthopaedic Association announced that: *Most surgeons are aware of what constitutes a proper relationship and what is a breach of the Association's code of conduct.* So far so good but the situation is that a duty of care to patients might be replaced by lucrative contractual arrangements with a provider whereby both parties enjoy benefits which supersede patients' best interests. The problem, of course, with codes of conduct between makers and doctors is that they are worthless without severe penalties for transgressions and effective surveillance of purchasing choices.

But it is not only prosthetic orthopaedics which encounters unethical temptations. Heart valves, hearing-aids, splints, neck braces, drainage-tubes, cardiac catheters, balloons, stents and a multitude of similar devices are being sold daily by companies who reward users according to the frequency of their choice of the device. In other words, misconduct is almost impossible to police outside of public hospitals as it is elsewhere. It is simply (perhaps an inappropriate word here) a matter of conscience.

'Crossing boundaries' — sexual exploitation of patients

Sexual relationships between doctors and patients have always created serious ethical conflict. In general, whether they are voluntary or involuntary on the part of a patient, they carry threats of deregistration and prosecution for doctors, even though mitigating factors may include a 'significant' period of time between a relationship and when the doctor was treating the patient. It has been suggested that five to ten percent of doctors persist in having sexual relations with current or past patients in breach of acceptable rules of conduct.

Reports from Australia and elsewhere suggest that the majority of offenders are male. Some figures suggest that psychiatrists offend twice as frequently as other doctors and many claim provocation by patients. Occasionally, these relationships evolve into conventional partnerships but, for the most part, unwelcome sexual advances by doctors are almost universally destructive of the professional relationship.

Cherrie Galletly published a paper with this title in the Medical Journal of Australia in 2004. It was provoked by the persistent reporting of such behaviour for as long as medical ethics have been discussed. Some offenders seem incurable. There is considerable public pressure for the most severe penalties to be imposed for offences which are usually regarded as clear violations of trust. On the other hand, an increasing informality in relationships between patients and doctors has been blamed for some 'random' violations. Homosexual offences seem much less frequent than heterosexual and there have been few reports of sexual molestation of children or the disabled.

Galletly lists some common but not always obvious danger-signals in medical relationships. They include discussion of a doctor's family and religious beliefs, admiring a patient's physical attributes, exchanging gifts, conspiratorial activity to deceive a third party, special scheduling of appointments, modified fee structures and making exceptions for attractive patients.

Moral values, rights and duties in medical treatment and research have roots traced back to ancient Greece but they are complicated by recent advances in innovative treatment which might increase the social awareness of human rights leading to resentment of the social positioning of doctors. Voluntary human experiments of all sizes and types have provoked the development of commissions for the protection of human subjects of medical research. End-of-life support, cloning, genetic testing, physician-assisted suicide, development of new and innovative medical products are ingredients of a continuous debate.

Organisations such as WHO, UNESCO and the International Association of Bio-ethics have been founded in the last 25 years to facilitate the exchange of information on these issues. In North America alone, there are more than 25 universities offering degrees in medical ethics and many medical schools include undergraduate courses in moral decision-making and responsible conduct in research.

So is Hippocrates relevant to the 21st century?

No one would argue with concepts of respect for duty, obligations and commitment. Notions of an individual's autonomy have been central to this tradition — the right to determine one's own fate and to live as one chooses, as long as that does not interfere with the rights of others. Some ethicists have promoted the principle of moral empiricism in which actions are judged primarily by their results. That is, if actions achieve good results for the greatest number of people, they are probably moral and justified, even if arguable. Central to all considerations of medical ethics has been an intuitive belief that if a student is taught well, he will do what is right — a view surely born more of hope than conviction.

Of course, proper acceptance of autonomy, attitudes of goodness, charity, mercy, justice and health for the disadvantaged are issues threaded through all ethical history but two central Hippocratic theses stand tall over all others — that nobody has the right to harm anybody else and that burdens and benefits should be spread evenly. All of those principles may come into play in a patient who is in profound coma and being kept alive mechanically but without expectation of recovery. The difficulties in decisions about disconnecting a life-support system are often raised. It presupposes that, by so doing, an irrecoverable patient can then be *allowed to die with dignity*. Obviously, families and doctors take advice and search their consciences about setting time-limits and exhausting all chances of even partial recovery.

A much more common conflict is: how much to explain to a gravely-ill patient when the whole truth may be so upsetting as to interfere with treatment programs? Families might request a doctor to conceal or soften the information which is given and many patients may die of an illness that had been more carefully explained to relatives than to the patient.

A maximally difficult problem is posed when a sentient patient elects to discontinue treatment, preferring to die while mentally competent and *in everyone's way*. While it is a doctor's duty to try to save and prolong life, healthcare systems might see their obligations differently when sustaining life is both enormously expensive and predictably futile.

Right-to-life

In the 1960s when birth-control pills first went on sale, the relative rights of the foetus and pregnant women also re-engaged the minds of doctors, ethicists and theologians. The US Supreme Court legalised abortion in 1973 and Canada followed suit in 1988, allowing it to be a confidential matter between a patient and her doctor. Ever since, the origin, meaning and definition of *personhood* have gone the rounds in Western societies.

Just when some headway seemed to be near, the 'morning-after' pill arrived. Unlike the original contraceptive pill, it involved the deliberate destruction of an already-fertilised egg within a few days of conception. Old questions arose again: When does life actually begin? Is this a form of euthanasia? The situation was exacerbated when RU-486, a drug which induced abortion of developed embryos up to two months of age, was marketed in Europe, Sweden and the US in 2000.

These various abortive procedures have aroused enormous debate about the *right-to-life*. Those in favour of abortion say it is always a private matter between a woman and her doctor and should be kept that way, free of harassment by anti-abortionists. Because RU-486 is not generally recognised by medical insurance schemes, unless a pregnancy results from rape or incest or endangers the life of the mother, the availability of this modern form of late contraception remains confined to the wealthier end of society.

Life-promotion

Infertility and the means of correcting it are important areas of medical ethics and doctors in family practices are asked initially to discuss procedures with many couples seeking advice. Specialised clinics offer measures which vary in their complexity, ethics, success-rates and invasion of the personal concepts of those involved. Artificial insemination, anonymous sperm or egg donation, donor privacy, entitlement of donors to parental rights, or even financial compensation, crowd the ethical scene.

In 1978, the first 'test-tube baby' was born from in vitro fertilisation [IVF] — the fertilisation of an egg in a laboratory before placing the primitive embryo in the prospective mother's uterus. Many variants of that technique have developed in the last 30 years. With its increased liability to multiple births, a secondary intervention may be needed to limit the number of surviving embryos.

The even more sensitive personal and ethical challenges of surrogate parenthood, where one or both partners do not contribute to the embryo, are matched in complexity only by questions about the disposal of fertilised eggs that are never implanted, or whose owner dies, or becomes incapacitated, or decides to generate no more children.

To compound these delicate problems, the advent of genetic testing 50 years ago made it possible to detect genetic defects in a foetus or embryo long before birth. It invited debate on the morality of using such genetic knowledge to end a pregnancy before it produced a child with substantial disability, if it survived at all. Similarly, some believe that 'unhealthy' IVF embryos discovered before implantation or gestation might best be discarded. That implies the possibility of acceptable 'designer' embryos while a slightly imperfect embryo might be unwanted. Increasingly, doctors and others are being asked to debate the profound ethical and practical aspects of 'tailor-made' babies.

Modern medicine has lately researched a different type of 'genetic engineering' by the in vitro manipulation of the parts of body-cells which carry the blueprint for inheritance. Experimentally, genes can be removed, modified and then inserted into the same or another cell, allowing their activity to then alter the very elements of life. The whole set of genes in the nucleus of every cell [its 'genome'] may be mapped to the extent that the bio-technology industry is hastening to get agreement to patent certain human genes, perhaps indefinitely — even if the ultimate function of those genes is presently unknown. Obviously, it is feared that gene-patenting could prevent the medical world generally from sharing knowledge about those genes and having equal access to them.

Cloning

In a process involving de-programming and re-programming of cell nuclei, scientists took the cell nucleus from an adult sheep's breast and used it to replace, in vitro, a cell nucleus of another sheep. The modified cell was then matured and put into a surrogate mother's uterus and carried to term. When Dolly [named after Dolly Parton because of her breast origin] was born, she was, in effect, an identical twin of her surrogate mother. She was born in 1997 and lived for six years. There was such widespread argument about the prospect of human cloning that President Clinton banned all Federal US funding for its research. Many other countries also prohibit human cloning by law but the technique continues to arouse fierce ethical and political debate.

Doctors' personal health risks

The advent of HIV-based AIDS 30 years ago starkly demonstrated the vulnerability of doctors to become infected with a deadly disease by contact with an infected patient. Many doctors refused to treat such patients, or even those who just might be infected, raising the questions of what basic rights does the doctor have and what can be done to protect him or her. Are they obliged to treat patients with a communicable and potentially fatal disease — an issue that had arisen during the plagues and deadly influenzas which swept Europe long ago?

And yet governments and some experts in ethics and law [even some surgeons] believe that no patient should suffer discrimination because of infection with HIV or other communicable diseases. There is no uniformity in the attitude of governments to this problem but, in many cases, it has been insisted that the unwilling doctor must either treat the patient or take urgent measures to find an alternative carer.

Experimentation

Regardless of how much animal testing may have been done, it is agreed that new drugs should be tested in human volunteers before release onto the market. If fully informed of the reasons for or against involvement, and the potential risks, people often choose to be included in 'clinical trials'. Patients are told that they won't know, to begin, if they have received a 'fake' substance [a placebo] or the active drug being tested for its benefits.

They should also know that the drug trial must try to show which effects of the test drug, either good or bad, are *real* — not just a result of patients *believing* they were receiving effective treatment. Later, those who were in the placebo group discover that they received no potentially useful treatment at all during the testing and some might have been disadvantaged by that delay. Of course, there are compensations offered to the participants in return, one of which is that they may be allowed prior access to any new and proven drug developed during their participation or later.

Completely opposite conditions applied in the WW2 experiments conducted by Nazi doctors on involuntary subjects, as were exposed during the Nuremberg trials between 1945 and 1949. There, twenty-three Nazi doctors were accused and 16 of them were judged guilty of extraordinary procedures that had no possible medical justification. Japanese doctors were similarly disciplined for grossly unethical procedures both during and after WW2. Disturbingly, US authorities have been accused of concealing the identity of some Japanese perpetrators in order to enhance their own understanding and to protect the *security* of both nations.

In the years following WW2, secret medical experimentation on uninformed subjects occurred when hundreds of pregnant US mothers were given a radioactive substance in order to investigate the amount of their iron stores. Similarly, children with developmental disabilities in a State hospital were deliberately infected with hepatitis in order to develop a vaccine against that disease. Worse still, cancer cells were injected into other unknowing patients to test their immune responses.

Most criticised of all, perhaps, was an experiment in Alabama, beginning in 1932. Researchers wanted to study the natural history of untreated syphilis for as many years as possible. To that end, although a cure for syphilis [penicillin] became available towards the end of the study period, a large number of syphilitic African-American men were not told of their diagnosis and received no treatment for syphilis until the investigation was finished or they had died because of their untreated disease.

Mortality and brain-death

Whatever the legislation and ethical argument, to decide when life has finally ended, what constitutes a reasonable quality of life and whether the patient, health system or courts should have ultimate authority in deciding life or death remain profoundly challenging confrontations for doctors. Above and beyond all these lofty principles, it is probably true to say that a new medical graduate's life is changed forever by the first experience of formally certifying the departure of another's life.

Since time began, death was accepted when there was a prolonged absence of pulse and breathing but, in the 1960s, technological advances in support-systems allowed doctors to artificially maintain life by those criteria almost indefinitely despite evidence of profound brain damage with widespread cell death. Doctors, families and institutions had to think about when brain-death has become irreversible, regardless of support systems for the rest of the body.

Generations of doctors have searched to find a way through the situation where life-support may no longer be justified on compassionate and economic grounds. Only that decision can open the gates to deciding who is eligible to donate tissues and organs to countless moribund patients who might have life as a result of transplantations.

In 1975, a US woman became permanently vegetative after an excessive dose of tranquilisers and alcohol. Eventually, her parents requested that she should be disconnected from life-support when they believed it would have been their daughter's wish. But hospital authorities could not agree and a long court battle followed. Ultimately the court agreed with the parents and their daughter was disconnected from her respirator.

Here is where ethical chaos began: she began to breathe spontaneously and lived another ten years though clinically 'brain-dead'. Nothing changed after disconnecting the respirator. Of course, the fact that she had no need for 'life-support' should have been identified long before the drama of court work. For her to die, something more 'active' was required, such as suspension of feeding, but nobody wanted to get into yet another tricky area of debate.

The Netherlands legalised *voluntary* euthanasia in 2000, provided that it had the full consent of the patient and all involved doctors. Similarly, voters in the state of Oregon voted in 1994 and 1997 to approve the prescription of lethal medications when requested by a mentally competent adult suffering in the final stages of a terminal illness but in most of North America, euthanasia remains illegal.

The 'Baby Doe' case issued yet another sort of challenge in the US in 1982. Who had the right to withhold treatment from a highly-dependent child, in this case one with Down's syndrome including a severe malformation affecting both breathing and swallowing? The parents were unwilling to preserve her life and refused to consent to a form of surgery that could have improved matters, at least temporarily. Without that treatment, the baby died six days later. President Reagan hastened the passage of legislation to prevent similar conflicts and doctors were relieved that they could then follow elementary, practical, surgical principles for potentially correctable 'structural' problems.

Definitions and 'jumping the gun'

After many deliberations flowing from the early period of heart transplantation, more refined and unarguable criteria of 'brain-stem' death were agreed on by the Royal [medical] Colleges of England in 1976. That concept was quite widely adopted throughout the world as a reliable and decent reflection of irrecoverability but there was no consensus. A major sticking point was and is whether irreversible 'cardiac' death should be enough to define the moment when organ harvesting might begin.

The unseemly, global scramble to get involved in heart transplantation meant that 107 transplants were carried out by 64 surgical teams in 24 countries during 1968. The results were generally poor. Some surgeons were ill-trained and lacked adequate support services. The matching of donors and recipients was not rigorous and there was a great deal still to be learned about after-care and the control of rejection.

Inevitably, religious groups have weighed into arguments concerning the temptation for surgeons to 'jump the gun' to obtain multiple, 'fresh' organs for distribution amongst several possible recipients. Pope Benedict has expressed this concern especially in terms of 'trafficking' in illegally obtained organs from living donors, related or otherwise to a recipient. In one US cardiac centre, hearts were taken for transplantation from brain-damaged newborns within a few minutes of certified cardiac death. There have certainly been widespread reservations about the assumption that brain-death defines whole-person death.

Clearly, there are no hard-and-fast rules yet agreed universally. The continuing arguments about brain-death or heart-death defining irreversible death show that these issues remain to be settled. They may remain so indefinitely despite rules being considered to be 'set-in-stone' 20 years ago. As late as October 2008 a Melbourne paediatrician claimed that the accepted legal interpretation of death [irreversible loss of function of brain or heart] was frequently ignored in order to obtain 'live' organs for donation within minutes of clinical 'death'. Others believe that current definitions are adequate in major institutions which have transplant programs.

The transfer of viable tissues or organs of one human to another provides great benefit to those who are disabled or doomed without that assistance. There may be a quarter of a million potential recipients in the world today awaiting some form of transplantation. Most of them die while on a waiting list because there are never enough tissues or organs to go around.

A major difficulty for doctors is to secure the consent of family members to remove organs from a dying but not yet dead donor. Another is to find living, mentally normal donors who are prepared to donate one of their *paired* organs such as a kidney. In some countries, organ and tissue harvesting has been legalised from all those who have **not** already specified their objection [such as on a driving licence] before reaching a state of impending and inevitable death.

Organs and tissues can also be *sold* on the understanding that a poor match or infective complication remains the sole responsibility of the recipient. More startling are reports from several countries that donor's *essential* and *non-essential* organs are being procured from both *willing* and *unwilling* donors. Willing donors are paid for their organs. If that means their death by donation of essential organs, their families are rewarded. Unwilling donors go unrewarded and die while the organ procurers charge recipients exorbitantly for fresh, made-to-measure organs. Anecdotally, many surgeons have been suspected of itinerant involvement in this financially-rewarding form of the transplantation industry.

More complex biologically has been the question of *xeno-transplantation* — using animal donations into humans, despite risks of rejection and transmission of animal diseases. Various procedures have been used to maximise the safety of transferring 'foreign' animal proteins such as occur in heart valves, tissue patches and blood vessels. Meantime, frantic efforts continue to construct animal donors who have been genetically modified to be closely compatible with humans.

Inevitably, these issues promote interest in the use of human *'stem-cells'* [primitive, all-purpose embryonic cells] to regenerate destroyed or diseased tissues in willing recipients. The various means of getting potentially ideal *embryonic* human stem cells, and the manipulations involved in their use, have produced some of the most vigorous ethical debates of all time. 'Is it morally acceptable to use tissues taken from a human embryo at all? Are stem cells equally useful if taken from the recipient, or another human, or even an animal?' These issues tax the ingenuity of patients, doctors, politicians and ethicists alike.

Added to the enormous costs of such experimentation are problems arising from the enlarging population of possible recipients in societies where life expectation is increasing and the costs of extended maintenance falls on taxpayers at large. *'End-of-life'* issues, therefore, intrude frequently into the daily landscape of all doctors, particularly those in busy clinical practice.

The donor wasn't dead!

Just when the definition of brain-death seemed a little closer to resolution, it was reported on June 11, 2008 that a confirmed organ donor without pulse or breathing after 90 minutes of cardiac arrest in a major French transplant hospital had 'awoken' spontaneously just as the transplant surgeons were preparing to remove his organs. The 'donor' was walking and talking at home a few weeks later.

Even more bizarre, ABC News, Australia, reported on August 19, 2008, that a 'stillborn', premature baby in Israel had been formally pronounced dead and had been in a hospital refrigerator for more than five hours before release to her parents for burial. They then discovered the child was moving and she was returned to intensive care. A hospital director explained that, '... when we don't know how to explain things ... we call it a miracle.'

Chapter 4

Christiaan Barnard and brain-death

Although Barnard sent the surgical world into a frenzy when he was the first to transplant a human heart into another human in Cape Town in 1967, he was by no means the first to attempt organ or tissue transplantation. Cosmas and Damian, early Christian twin martyrs, were shown in many paintings and illustrations to be grafting a leg from a recently dead, black man onto the amputation stamp of a white man.

In each depiction of this procedure, the patient was shown lying quietly with angels at his side, and another holding the amputated white leg. Whatever the outcome, the twins were revered as miracle workers and marched swiftly into the annals of transplant history until they were tortured and beheaded in 303AD, presumably for a form of malpractice ... no doubt a serious warning for surgeons of the 21st century.

In 1905, Alexis Carrel, and Charles Guthrie transplanted a puppy's heart into an adult dog's neck. The recipient dog with two hearts survived for nearly three hours before dying, presumably, from acute rejection of the foreign organ. Others soon attempted similar operations with similar results.

Norman Shumway and Richard Lower were busily refining their techniques of heart transplantation in dogs at Stanford University Hospital in Palo Alto, California in the 1950s. When the problems of rejection were reduced significantly, they were confident that surgeons would be able to use healthy human hearts from doomed victims of other diseases to replace failing hearts.

In late December, 1959, San Francisco's media breathlessly reported that *a young Stanford surgeon* [Lower] *has successfully transplanted a living heart from one dog to another.* From then, the season had opened for an all-out assault on the problems of controlling rejection which is universal when one creature's tissues are transplanted into another. Across the world, and particularly in North America, surgeons were practising transplantation on animals of various species, all hoping to be the first to reach a stage when they might repeat the procedure with humans. Not all were completely scrupulous and some cut surgical corners to get ahead of the next surgeon.

Amongst those besotted with the challenge was Christiaan Barnard who had performed the first kidney transplant in South Africa in 1959. He had also transplanted many dog hearts though none survived. There was much exchange of information between the various international surgical departments, particularly of the complex issues of controlling rejection, an inflammatory response provoked by the foreign proteins of someone else's organ.

Lower had been legitimately 'poached' from Stanford by the Medical College of Richmond, Virginia and visitors like Barnard, unable to conceal their infatuation with the prospect of joining the ranks of distinguished surgical scientists, watchfully 'stalked' Richmond, San Francisco and other North American clinics where the latest information was available.

Certification of death

Once again, crucial to the progress of cardiac transplantation history was the fundamental prerequisite to extend and refine the criteria of death to justify the removal of an organ like the heart without which life was impossible. Simply, there arose again the need for agreement about the criteria of 'irrecoverable death'. That meant an acceptance that the donor's brain would never work again and the beating heart was redundant in a physiological sense.

While centres around the world were seeking accord on these issues and were rapidly approaching the point of scientifically matching a brain-dead donor to a moribund recipient, Shumway and Lower hesitated just long enough to be sure that their techniques of rejection-control were good enough to justify the procedure. Suddenly and without notice, Barnard performed the first human heart transplantation in Cape Town on December 3, 1967, shortly after a final visit to see Shumway's and Lower's work.

The surgical world was catapulted into a state of shock. Barnard immediately became known as the *film star surgeon*, adored by a berserk, global press which he adored in return. The downside was that many believed that he had spied on Shumway and Lower whose years of painstaking research had laid the foundations for a human transplant. Barnard had then snatched the triumph from them at the last minute for which many believed that Barnard was an arrogant stuntman.

Unseemly haste?

The race then became a violent competition to see who would do something different or more stunning, using whichever donor seemed possibly useful (human or animal) in patients of whatever age and in what numbers. All over the world, conventional principles of medical integrity and conduct were being challenged. The definition of 'death' remained a worry but, increasingly, there was a temptation to bend rules progressively on the ground that it was essential to be able to procure donor hearts which were healthy and, above all, fresh. Alternatively, large animal hearts might prove useful, at least while awaiting a human donor.

Barnard's first transplant patient lived for 18 days before he died from infection produced by the rejection-control drugs which he required. But by then the precise details of matching and immune management that had been worked out so carefully by Shumway and Lower in hundreds of animal experiments were becoming known and available worldwide.

By then, the charismatic Barnard was enjoying the admiration of the world. He travelled widely and neglected his marriage, family and surgical reputation. For many, this was a time of reckless rivalry, flagrant media manipulation and self-promotion. Not only surgeons became involved in the global scramble. Hospitals, cardiologists, technicians, politicians and whole cities developed rivalries which were hitherto unknown. In one angry outburst, Barnard rejected a suggestion that the donor for his first transplant may not have been brain-dead by all reasonable criteria at the time.

Inevitably, Shumway and Lower were appalled that they had been 'pipped at the post' by a surgeon whose experimental experience was negligible compared with theirs'. Shumway was awaiting a suitable donor for a willing recipient at the very moment when Barnard had pounced onto the surgical stage. Just two weeks before Barnard's extravaganza, Shumway reported that *we think the way is clear for trial of human heart transplantation.* The personal relationships between Shumway, Lower and Barnard had been fractured forever.

What Barnard's legacy might have been had he not succumbed to the temptations that ultimately ruined him, nobody will ever know. His first marriage in 1948 produced a son who took his own life. In 1969, he married a glamorous young woman with whom he had two children. In 1988 he married for the third time, this time to a young model and had two children with her. That marriage lasted two years before she left him, taking the children with her. He was shattered.

In October 1975, it was already apparent that Barnard's status amongst many of his surgical contemporaries had long since collapsed. When 500 leading cardiac surgeons and cardiologists attended an international congress on cardiac surgery in Detroit in that year, Barnard was apparently not invited. His was only one of many, famous, cardiac surgical names damaged in one way or another. Many others destroyed their reputations trying to exceed his fame.

Barnard retired from cardiac surgery in 1983 with a diagnosis of rheumatoid arthritis affecting his hands. He soon became imbued with anti-ageing research. His reputation suffered further in 1986 when he promoted a very expensive skin cream alleged to control ageing. It was soon withdrawn from the market as a useless product. He then involved himself in an organisation in Switzerland exploring a controversial rejuvenation therapy which was also shown to be useless.

Shumway finally forgave Barnard who, by then, had not only lost his looks from massive facial surgery for cancer but, also, his three wives, his children, much of his professional reputation and all of his glory: *I now look more like the elephant man than the handsome guy who was once voted one of the world's five greatest lovers by Paris Match,* he wrote.

Barnard's brother surgeon, Marius, confessed his disenchantment with much of heart transplantation when he wrote as follows: *There are three reasons why the heart transplant became such a massive 20th century story. 1. Where was it done? In Cape Town, in the days of apartheid. 2. Two: Who did it? We were not Denton Cooley or Michael DeBakey. We were not Lord Brock in London or Norman Shumway at Stanford. We were just ordinary guys — and some of us, especially Chris, had good personalities in public. We were upfront and we weren't too bad looking. We were kind of poor — my monthly salary was $400 then. When people heard we came from this small Afrikaner town ... it was even more romantic but the biggest thing was number three: the heart. Who were the pioneers of kidney transplantation?* [Marius named three celebrated pioneers]. *No ordinary person knows their names* [today]. *But ask them who did the first heart transplant and they knew: 'Chris Barnard'.*

I just think it's sad that the only claim to fame that we have is not scientific — it's just that we did it first. Like Roger Bannister ran the first four-minute mile. So what? Everyone runs it in three minutes or so now. The first man on the moon? To hell with him! But people always need a name. And so, with a heart transplant, they got one: Chris Barnard. I think, in the end, the world got what it wanted.

Shortly after Barnard died from asthma in Cyprus in September 2001, Norman Shumway said this about him: *He did make a hugely significant contribution to heart transplantation. What he did with brain-death should never be forgotten ... Barnard made the use of brain-dead victims for organ transplantation an acceptable concept. Of course, he and I didn't see much of each other ... the last time we met, it was June 2000 in Paris. He had this carcinoma of the nose, so his whole nose had been removed and grafts had been taken from his cheeks to build a new nose. Honest to God, I didn't even recognise him. I felt so sorry for him because I knew what looking like that did to him.*

Norman Shumway also died of cancer on February 10, 2006 at the age of 83. Two years earlier he was asked again about the disappointment of losing the race to transplant the first human heart. He replied: *Maybe it was a blessing that we weren't the first. We had enough trouble anyway dealing with the press and all that hoo-hah. Boy, we had plenty of trouble. So maybe, in the end, it all worked out for the best.* Even a man as imperturbable and gracious as Shumway must have found that compromise even a little painful.

Chapter 5

Crimes and punishments

One often hears that there is need for an analysis of how doctors are *'made'*, what is the nature of the medical hierarchy and where does the power of the profession lie. Understanding ethical conduct and performance probably relies on examining how the profession came to exist, the motives of the pioneers and, most of all, what causes men and women to *want* to work where immense humanity is expressed alongside risk of failure, constant envy, criticism, disillusionment and even persecution.

Why would any individual want to practise medicine when he or she might sooner or later be accused of having a deep flaw in character leading to unacceptable conduct?

In no other profession apart from holy orders are inappropriate patterns of behaviour so viciously publicised. We are all made aware daily of doctors' dishonesty, their intentional or inadvertent harming of patients, sexual harassment and involvement in fraud or substance abuse. No wonder it is often suggested that the medical profession is preoccupied by protecting itself from criticism and humiliation — as if that attitude was unique to doctoring.

Whether or not medical practitioners fear retaliatory criticism from other health practitioners because of envy or rivalry, and risk libel suits if they 'dob-in' a colleague for misconduct, as we have seen earlier, there is a much larger number of complaints aimed at doctors every year from other quarters. The vast majority are made by patients and later found to be fairly inconsequential. Nonetheless, an attack on 'competence', in any sense of that word, is a potentially mortal blow to a doctor's self-esteem, reputation and practice. The stigma easily becomes permanent and threatens employment. Few, if any, alternative occupations are readily available. And yet, regardless of a continuing shortage of all health workers [apart from psychological 'counsellors'], complaints against doctors and nurses increase by the day, regardless of their substance.

At the worst end of the scale, to be charged with a 'criminal' act severely damages a doctor's reputation forever. After only seven such charges in the UK for 120 years, 13 have been brought within the last 20 years. The usual claim is one of 'manslaughter', with or without an element of intent, and with criminal prosecution being the outcome. No doubt that extreme attitude rests uneasily with less aggressive legal practitioners and doctors but no comparison has been made with lawyers' deviance, obfuscation, errors and omissions.

On the other hand, a medical authority from the UK reminded us that *many* [medical] *errors occur by a combination of circumstances often out of control of the individual* [doctor]. Nonetheless, legal systems avidly seek to identify any instance of medical misadventure where damage and blame can possibly be established. Society demands that any untoward outcome of a medical procedure must mean that there is a punishable 'fault'. Thus, as has been discussed above in cases of 'post-traumatic stress disorder' [PTSD], society's hurts may sometimes be addressed effectively only by finding somebody to blame and then by being compensated financially.

In another context referred to earlier, Cyclone Katrina in New Orleans in 2005 produced a situation when doctors mercifully killed mortally-ill patients who had no hope of evacuation to safe places. One specialist said that, if one dose had not killed her patient, she would give another. She did not regard her actions as murder or manslaughter. She said: *This was compassion. They would have been dead within hours if not days.* She finally fled the hospital instead of also being killed by the armed looters.

This experience has forced her to take a second look at the nature of triage: those obviously likely to survive get maximum help; those needing urgent care with a reasonable chance of survival get next priority; those who are inevitably dying and unsalvageable are helped on their way with maximum humanity and adequate narcosis.

But euthanasia remains illegal in Louisiana! So where does that leave conventional medical ethics and arguments against euthanasia? How does it lead doctors through the agonies of some decision-making throughout medical life? Most importantly, how do their decisions compare in gravity and responsibility with those of lawyers, politicians, corporations, priests and the man in the street?

→

As a uniquely vulnerable and targeted professional group, doctors are very easy targets for blame by what is called a 'free' press. It is unusual for a week to pass without a media report of medical error or misconduct, usually as a headline with photographs. It may be implied that doctors perpetrate some of the greatest threats that humanity can face. A well-performed though unsuccessful surgical operation may be made to appear more important in human affairs than the horrifying, endemic wars of Africa with their ongoing millions of casualties.

While the daily media are preoccupied with destruction and freely disseminate errors of fact and unbalanced opinions, those are overlooked in their relentless pursuit of doctors. Nonetheless, many polls show that the population at large trusts doctors more than it trusts any other professional group — certainly more than lawyers, politicians, journalists and priests. While no individual or institution is secure from criticism, away from the perennial 'scandal and horror' headlines the public generally thinks that their doctors serve them well.

Of course, untoward events are inevitable in medical matters. They vary according to the nature of the doctor-group involved, the pathology treated, geographic location, support services, consultant availability, hospital access and, with specialists, the nature of their work. It should go without saying that procedures conducted by a surgeon whose principal, and chosen, activity involves the intricacies of the heart or brain, large acute trauma, extensive cancer, the very elderly and very young and complex obstetrics will have more disappointing outcomes than other practitioners. It is part and parcel of their chosen work and they do not shrink from it unless litigation risks become totally destructive of practice.

Of course, there have always been 'bad' doctors — arrogant, drunken, immoral, lazy and dishonest. We all accept that they have variable skills, manners and rectitude, just as all humanity has the same imperfections. To expect otherwise is unrealistic but we seem to be surprised by that. Doctoring is an inherently risky activity with results that are often immediately apparent. It is quite unlike the activities of journalism or law or financial institutions which may do enormous harm with no correction or recompense offered or considered necessary.

But it is quite inevitable that prolific and ugly media stories, without fair and proper analysis, must hasten the point where there is a loss of professional morale, early retirement of competent doctors and nurses and diminished resources — particularly in remote and semi-remote locations. Recent government health proposals appear to overlook or pretend that these attritional factors do not exist, despite their being evident for generations and worsening as human health resources shrink.

The purely commercial effects of the rabid hunting of doctors by the media and lawyers for evidence of negligence when none may exist are that health workers are increasingly loaded with expensive insurance costs which are inevitably passed on to consumers. Protection is needed even against minor litigation. While relative peace of mind comes at a great cost for doctors, nothing can cure the deep, personal damage that an unjustified claim of negligence inflicts.

None of these comments is meant to defend explicit shortcomings in medical workers. We have already seen and will see again later the nature and quantity of their deficiencies. Clearly, scrutiny of their activities is a proper part of their licensing but it is fair to say that, within the current climate of antipathy promoted by the media and legal profession, it will continue to be difficult or impossible to maintain adequate health delivery in all countries, including the most affluent. Already, more than one-half of all primary-care doctors in Australia are foreign graduates who are especially vulnerable to criticism. Once a community loses confidence in the individual values and capabilities of its medical professionals, it becomes a more dangerous place to live.

In many ancient medical publications there have been remarkably similar views expressed, if not frank warnings, that acts of medical misconduct could result in penalties — divine, secular or both. Hundreds of years BC, Hippocrates was imbued with a sense of equality between physicians and priests. Philanthropy, generosity, goodness, mercy, purity and holiness shaped his principles of proper behaviour. These recurring themes have spread across many boundaries of civilisation ever since — all apparently intuitive and without prior collaboration.

Of course Hippocrates was critical of deliberate wrongdoing, mischief-making, secret transactions, improper sexual relationships, procuring abortion or euthanasia and medical undertakings in which the practitioner was not expert. He implied that the transgression of these boundaries might preclude 'recognition' of a medical practitioner — in effect, his or her 'registration' to practise.

In the first millennium, Hebrew, Chinese and Moslem writers promoted very similar principles for medical pupils who were seeking professional acceptance and some form of registration. Chinese medical virtues included determination and mercy, sexual continence, equal service to rich and poor, generosity, selflessness, discretion, modesty and care in prescribing. Greed, lust, seeking riches and procuring abortion, would surely be punished by God. Surgically speaking, 'breaking open the flesh of man with an iron instrument or searing by fire' could be justified only by great contemplation — perhaps an early warning or admonition for aggressive surgeons. How effectively war surgery can be conducted with such strictures is imponderable.

Chapter 6

Pitfalls and penalties of practice

W hile most doctors are ethical and skilled, some may fail to achieve what they set out to do despite their best efforts and others may not follow acceptable standards of practice. Whatever the reason — inadvertence, inattention, illness, isolation, inexperience or confronting an extraordinary situation never experienced before — they may cause harm. Intent to do harm must be extremely rare but the result for a patient may be the same as that resulting from the best care possible under all the existing circumstances.

However experienced the doctor may be, none can guarantee success because, almost by definition, no action involving a patient's anatomy, physiology and pathology can ever be without any risk. To professionally touch another's body or mind — their most prized and personal possessions — constitutes a remarkable but very necessary invasion of a patient's privacy, however trivial or conventional or legitimate it may seem to the doctor and patient. But in all things, the ultimate boundary is that every doctor is expected to act in the same way as *any other reasonably-qualified and prudent practitioner* [would do] *in a similar situation.* Of course, that proviso assumes that a *similar situation* can be defined without too many assumptions or prejudice.

Litigation

Bringing a doctor before a court for a medical error is a fairly recent notion. Ancient Europe allowed doctors immunity from punishment for almost any wrong they did. When the Great Plague had killed a third of the population of England in the 14th century, doctors were blamed for failing to prevent or to cure it. Soon after, an irrational or ignorant judge ruled that a doctor could be liable to complaint if he failed to cure a patient within a 'reasonable' period of time. And so the earliest known malpractice judgement surfaced and created an absurd precedent for all time.

In the early 19th century, a US doctor removed a woman's breast for what he believed was a tuberculous infection. When the patient later bled to death for no known reason, a court found that the doctor should withhold his bill and compensate the husband for the loss of his wife's companionship. Thereafter, any reasonably justified penalty might be imposed on a doctor if a judge felt so inclined, usually with no appeal allowed. The stage had been set for a massive and almost totally uninformed legal invasion of medical practice with far-reaching penalties in costs and sense.

On every day of 1990, nearly one thousand malpractice complaints were brought against US doctors. Obstetricians and gynaecologists in New York State were being sued four times more often than their colleagues in Canada and Great Britain. The reasons for the excess rate of claims included a general recognition that American doctors were wealthy, that they were reluctant to treat patients who were not medically insured and, as still assumed today, that successful medical care was everybody's God-given right. At the same time, legal claims against doctors were encouraged by 'contingency' arrangements where no-win for the patient meant no-pay for the lawyer. So, the flood-gates of litigation were widely opened and impossible to close, despite the progressive costs of 'defensive' medical practice.

Lawsuits are not initiated in most cases of alleged medical malpractice. They are either defended by a doctor's insurer, or private financial settlements are made. Of those that do proceed to court, only about five percent ever reach a verdict and doctors are much more likely to 'win' than the patients who are suing.

The greatest risk of litigation arises when fully-informed consent is not obtained before a medical intervention. However managed, serious difficulties are inevitable in the case of emergencies, extreme pathology, in treating the under-aged, the infirm, those of unsound-mind, of certain religions and conscientious objectors. There, the doctor must rely on all reasonable measures to inform the patient and next of kin of his best advice. It may be that court orders are sought to circumvent irrational risk-taking by patients and their families.

A predictable limitation on claims and damage verdicts had to be found in the extreme climate of litigation which boomed in the mid-1980s in all Western countries. Insurance premiums became so high that doctors lost interest in continuing medical practice or moved across state borders or overseas to less litigious areas of practice. As mentioned above, 'defensive' medical practice means that repeated, costly tests are ordered to avoid being accused of shoddy investigation of even trivial complaints. Hence, the costs of modern medical technology have become an intolerable burden on the economies of most developed countries while the providers of that technology have prospered beyond all expectations.

Where are medical ethics heading?

While reliance on the Hippocratic Oath is generally regarded as a reliable and fundamental guide for physicians and other health workers, some authorities have questioned the need for medical ethics at all. It has been suggested that ethicists and philosophers are intervening for their own practice, curiosity and benefit in matters which are part and parcel of the natural evolution of acceptable and appropriate practice — implying a more or less empiric process. Others take the more pragmatic view that what is accepted as appropriate to Western medicine may have little relevance to the chaotic deprivation of under-developed countries.

New medical developments present very knotty questions for all doctors to ponder, whether or not they are asked them. HIV/AIDS and lung cancer are diseases which, in some sense, might be regarded as self-inflicted. Does that make a difference to how they are treated? Who should be tested for HIV anyway? How does the doctor tell new Western parents that circumcision is a good idea because it probably reduces HIV infection rates in Africans? But is circumcision an improper assault on a baby boy's human rights anyway? How can the stigma and discrimination associated with HIV be avoided? On the other hand, the recognition that Human Papilloma Virus (HPV) affecting teenagers and young women causes cancer means that a young, secretive teenager might best be advised privately to insist on a condom during sexual activity. But should her parents be told and, if so, by whom?

The multiplicity of difficulties confronting doctors and the patients who are affected by these decisions suggests that medical ethics may have diminishing relevance. Certainly, most people would not want to know of the baffling problems involving a doctor, let alone want to carry the responsibility for giving advice in these matters. Those decisions may produce great personal anguish for a doctor but, if medical advice is less than frank and luck goes against the doctor, highly destructive accusations of negligence may inevitably follow.

Chapter 7

Controlling bodies

Numerous institutions have been established to regulate and monitor medical practices by individuals and institutions. Those mentioned in this chapter vary in their mechanisms and penalties but their intentions are uniformly good and practical with the patients' best interests at heart.

The American College of Surgeons [ACS] is a conservative organisation of overt integrity. Its fellowship is highly respected and jealously guarded. Shortly after the College's inception in 1913, it empowered a Central Judiciary Committee [CJC] to be concerned, in the first place, with reducing '*fee splitting*' and '*itinerant surgery*' which were prevalent at the time. Since then, the CJC has dealt with all forms of licensing, behavioural disorders and varieties of unprofessional conduct amongst members.

In the last decade or so, the ACS has been severely challenged by members without adequate credentials acting as 'expert' witnesses in court proceedings, some against other College Fellows, so that it has had to clearly delineate the essential qualifications of an expert. That is: to have current, active involvement in the type of procedure being considered and to avoid the temptation to 'sell' flexible opinions to the highest bidder. (See Chapter 10, Case 1.)

Disciplinary actions include admonition, censure, probation, suspension and expulsion. The grounds for adverse judgement are almost identical to those adopted by all other Western medical institutions and closely resemble those set out by Hippocrates and ancient Muslim, Hebrew and Chinese ethicists.

Of 104 penalties imposed by the ACS between 1993 and 2003, 40% of disciplined doctors were placed on probation, 30% were expelled, 20% were suspended and the remainder were admonished or censured. A right of appeal is not automatic. The most severe penalty, expulsion, means that a College membership certificate is forfeited. Unless expulsion is later reversed, the disowned surgeon cannot behave as if he or she remains a Fellow of the ACS or function in any way in a College program.

The following CJC synopses relate to typical examples of offences and penalties decided in recent times. They are indistinguishable from those of other Western tribunals. A concentration of 'fairness' is evident:

1. A surgeon was charged with abuse of both alcohol and cannabis. His registration was suspended and he was ordered intensive residential treatment with no possible return to practice until the program was successfully completed. After some delay, he underwent private treatment. He could not return to practice until he had demonstrated recovery from 'excessive use of alcohol, drugs, chemicals or any other types of material'. After multiple reviews by the College and his demonstration of rehabilitation, full surgical Fellowship privileges were restored.

2. A surgeon's licence was suspended following allegations of substance abuse, poor standards of care and the unlicensed practice of medicine. He was found guilty on 19 counts of unprofessional conduct related to marijuana, alcohol, pethidine, morphine and cocaine during more than five years. He was found guilty of gross and repeated negligence in two cases and one had resulted in a patient's death. When he failed to respond to multiple invitations to attend the College for discussions, he was expelled.

3. A surgeon questioned the evidence given by another surgeon acting as an expert witness in a law suit. The accused was said to have shown bias in his opinion, not thoroughly reading the relevant medical records and making misleading remarks. He did not respond to College requests for his comments on the accusations. An advisory body considered that he had violated College standards for giving expert testimony. Following further investigation and testimonials, he was admonished but retained his Fellowship.

4. Another 'expert witness' was alleged to have violated College rules by giving evidence while not actively practising in the speciality concerned. His views were said to be unsupported by medical literature and not impartial. Because other specialty groups were also investigating the accused for the same complaint, the College investigation was postponed indefinitely. The accused retains his Fellowship.

5. A surgeon was accused of acting as an expert witness in a complaint about a hernia operation, although he had not performed that procedure for more than ten years. Some of his evidence was considered to have been inaccurate, misleading and unsubstantiated. The accused submitted a personal and legal response to the allegations. Review of all available evidence led to the recommendation that no further action should be taken.

6. An excessive number of complications following surgery for obesity suggested that a surgeon did not provide an acceptable standard of care and a hospital had suspended him from operating. He was also suspended by the College for six weeks and then placed on probation with limited practice conditions for the next seven and a half years. He is required to have a mentor and advisor present at his next 100 cases and to provide complete records for review by the College. He was fined $25,000.00 and asked to suspend internet advertising. The surgeon remains under restrictions.

The US State Medical Boards oversee alternative as well as conventional medicine. In 1912, all States combined to collect and distribute information about disciplinary actions taken against doctors and to record details on a comprehensive database. Initially, the database was only available to US entities but, with increased public demand for information about doctors, it was opened in 2001 to international licensing authorities including Canada, England, Australia and New Zealand.

The UK General Medical Council examines doctors' activities in the interest of public safety and confidence. Since it was created in 1858, there has been much sporadic dissatisfaction expressed about its administration and decision making. It has now accepted the innovation of allowing general practitioners working for the National Health Service to remove certain patients from their allocated lists, such as for violent, threatening or abusive behaviour.

The Australian Health Practitioner Regulation Agency [AHPRA], otherwise known as the Australian Medical Board, was established as a Federal authority on July 1, 2010. It consists of most of the medical boards of the States and Territories whose rules are essentially interchangeable. From July 2010, registration in any State or Territory will be recognised nationally to enable rapid, universal and full exchange of information between those areas. The board will issue annual reports about individual doctors and events. Previously, the now incorporated NSW Medical Board, for example, received complaints from patients, other members of the public, medical and other health care professionals and various professional institutions about doctors' behaviour. AHPRA's scrutiny of doctors' CVs particularly concerns those applying for registration from a foreign country.

The NSW Medical Board [NSWMB, now included within the AHPRA] was originally constituted in 1838 to define the qualifications of medical practitioners. A register of approved practitioners, with their signatures and photographs, was published annually in the NSW Government Gazette for the information of coroners, magistrates and the public at large. There was also a jealously guarded register of specialists.

A truly disciplinary 'tribunal' was later established, sitting in open court with legal representations. A guilty practitioner could be reprimanded, suspended or deregistered. Not only did it later confer grades of registration but it also determined the conditions of registration of errant doctors and overseas medical graduates. The AHPRA will continue to issue annual reports which are in the public domain.

The NSW Board had become an independent statutory authority in 1986. Its major responsibilities, now administered by the AHPRA, were the registration of doctors, the counselling of medical students and the enforcement of standards of practice. It set out to maximise protection of the public through an ethical 'Code of Professional Conduct', modelled on the General Medical Council [UK] guidelines of 2000.

The NSW Board previously worked in a system of 'co-regulation' with the Health Care Complaints Commission [HCCC]. As that will continue, all complaints are assessed by both bodies, regardless of which receives the first notification, and the Commission will, presumably, prosecute complaints referred to a tribunal. A Code of Professional Conduct is relevant to all bodies which have a role in overseeing 'proper and ethical conduct by a registered doctor'. To ensure rapid dissemination of doctors' registration records throughout Australia, the AHPRA's national register of all medical doctors and other health professionals in Australia is now available. (Those safety and disciplinary functions remain in the province of the **NSW Medical Council**.)

Historically, the NSW Medical Practice Amendment Act 2008 covered issues such as mandatory and protected reporting of misconduct, emergency protective powers, conditional registration, professional standards procedures, mandatory indemnity insurance for registration and special conditions for temporary registration of short-term visiting medical educators. New cosmetic surgery and advertising guidelines are amongst recent developments. It is unable to verify a doctor's claims of expertise based on an entire professional profile. Similar functions and limitations are expected within the new AHPRA.

NSW Medical Tribunals: Sitting as a District Court with a judge, two doctors and another person empanelled, tribunals have the power to impose whatever penalties they think fit. Here is a list of examples of the vast range of unacceptable conduct that has been evaluated in recent years:

Abandonment of skill, judgement and care; alteration of clinical records; fraud; attended at hospital under influence of alcohol; breach of child protection conditions; breach of AVO [Apprehended Violence Order]; breach of limited practice conditions; inadequate capacity to practise medicine; cognitive deficits; dishonestly purchasing wholesale drugs without a licence; non-disclosure to a medical board; failure to keep adequate drug register; failure to have authorisation to prescribe certain drugs; fraudulent use and distribution of prescriptions; inappropriate prescribing of drugs of dependence and addiction; physical and mental impairment; addiction to deleterious drugs; improper conduct; inappropriate actions at a patient's home; inappropriate prescription of anabolic steroids; indecent assault on patients; making false statements to The Health Insurance Commission; possession of child pornography; inappropriate social and physical contact with patient; concealment of alcohol dependence; unlimited, experimental drug prescribing for addicts; possession of prohibited and unlicensed firearms; rude and insensitive comments to patients; prescribing from medical practices which doctor did not attend; professional misconduct [various types]; gratuitous religious instruction during consultation; refusal to admit past misconduct [indecent assault]; self-administration of illicit drugs; sexual misconduct; unsatisfactory professional conduct.

The NSWMB's annual report of 2006-2007 referred to 1155 complaints received in that year, mostly to do with aspects of doctors' competence and conduct. Defects in communication and practice administration comprised the rest. Of 149 complaints referred for investigation, 66% required no further action or only advice and warning to the doctor. The rest were referred for explicit discipline by a Professional Standards Committee or a Medical Tribunal. One quarter of those doctors were deregistered. Others had conditions imposed on their style of practice, or reprimands.

The NSW Health Care Complaints Commission [HCCC] was established in 1993 to target errant health-care professionals, particularly medical doctors. It may refer matters of discipline to the NSWMB, to the Optometrists Board, the Physiotherapist Registration Board, the Nurses and Midwives Board or the Psychologists Registration Board. It apparently anticipates having jurisdiction over chiropractors, osteopaths, dental boards and technicians, optical dispensers, pharmacists and podiatrists. It casts, therefore, a very broad net in its investigative powers which it shares with the Medical Board.

For 15 years, its foundation chief, Merrilyn Walton, conducted many enquiries into doctors' behaviour and published widely on ethical practice, standards of care and patients' rights. Under her administration, the HCCC was variously described, with very little explanation, as either too lenient or too harsh in its pursuit of certain aspects of medical practice. Inevitably, Walton had her critics but she has been greatly admired for her accomplishments. Presently, she has an associate professorial post at Sydney University where her health interests continue.

The NSW Clinical Excellence Commission [CEC] was established in 2004 to *'promote and support improved clinical care, safety and quality across the NSW health system ... to build confidence in health care ... [making it] better and safer for patients and a more rewarding work place'.* Its key functions are to monitor the performance of public health organisations and their staff and to *report directly to the Minister for Health*. It is not directly concerned with particular doctors except when their actions may affect the performance of an institution. It examines matters requiring investigation in order to make the public health system work better. Essentially, it manages 'incidents' which threaten patient comfort, care and safety without imparting 'spin' to its reports to government.

In its 2005-2006 report, the CEC recorded 125,000 'notifications' of problems encountered in major public health institutions. Thirty percent of those notifications did not relate to actual patient care. Of the 70% that did, only 21% produced some degree of *harm* to patients and, of those, 3.6% resulted in *serious harm or death*.

No doubt, the various regulatory bodies have developed from imperatives to establish tighter controls over every aspect of medical care. For example, in public hospitals there are constant on-line systems for transfer of information about mishaps in the wards and operating theatres to a central hospital body. From there, information is disseminated to a health department, a medical board, the HCCC, the CEC, the Police or the Attorney-General.

The Australian Medical Council (AMC) describes itself as *'an independent national standards body for medical education and training. (Its purpose) is to ensure that standards of education, training and assessment of the medical profession promote and protect the health of the Australian Community'*. Thus, it assesses educational factors and foreign graduates who wish to practise in Australia, advises the Federal Government and others on registration and medical standards.

→

Clearly, there is a considerable degree of overlap between multiple Australian regulatory organisations. Some have a specific type of responsibility inherent in their charter and there is an inevitable degree of repetition in their published aims and responsibilities but that implies no necessary criticism of the governance that each body exercises according to its perceived responsibility. It is not yet entirely clear whether the combined surveillance by these bodies has added substantially to individual and overall patient and professional satisfaction. How the advent of the AMB (AHPRA) will affect these various bodies remains to be seen but it should go a long way towards improving the facility of data-transfer between states and territories.

Regardless of the number of such organisations, it seems that none has complete, if any, detailed knowledge of any doctor's ongoing, professional experience. Clearly that is an undesirable state of affairs. It is interesting to read in Brad Crouch's report in the South Australian *Sunday Mail* of December 13, 2009 that many eminent doctors have fiercely resisted all demands by the Royal Adelaide Hospital management and state health department to officially verify their credentials by providing certified copies of their primary medical degrees, postgraduate qualifications and curriculum vitae on the grounds of their preoccupation with busy practices and the inconvenience of complying.

Chapter 8

Medical experiments

Nuremberg

Nazi concentration camps were not quarantine stations of foreign nationals. They were places of systematic neglect and extermination. Medical and psychiatric staff were available but no medical assistance was provided to inmates. Between 1946 and 1947, Nuremberg became notorious as the scene of trials in which Nazi war criminals were brought before international military tribunals.

In examining the medical services of the Third Reich, 23 defendant doctors were put on trial. Most had worked for the German state. One suicided before sentencing, three were acquitted and 20 were found guilty of war crimes and crimes against humanity. Their leader, Karl Brandt, and 11 others were executed. Seven were imprisoned for periods of 15 years-to-life.

In his opening address at the Nuremberg Trials of Nazi doctors, a senior prosecutor summarised their extraordinary conduct by remarking that: *A nation which deliberately infects itself with poison will inevitably sicken and die. Germany was converted into an infernal combination of lunatic asylum and charnel house. The crimes were the result of sinister doctrines which sealed the fate of Germany, shattered Europe and left the world in ferment.*

Brandt was 32 years of age when he was appointed by Hitler to head the 'Office for Scientific and Medical Research'. He was in charge of a 'Euthanasia Program' to exterminate those of unsound body, mind or beliefs. His medical credentials for that appointment are unknown. His group abrogated every medical ethic in its involvement in the design and administration of concentration camps, the investigation and determination of ethnic superiority and inferiority and the conduct of living-human experimentation. None of the investigations could reasonably have been justified.

Collectively, the trial accounts make unbearable reading despite much of the language being sufficiently scientific to obscure the awful clinical details. Terrified individuals died in agony under the cold eyes of doctors and scientists who designed bizarre protocols, and then observed and recorded minute details of their manner of death.

The obscenity of Nazi medical experiments has been revealed by these verbatim abstracts of correspondence made available by The Jewish Internet Consortium. The shorthand style reflects the pragmatism of operators:

- *Letter to Brandt November 2, 1942: 150 skeletons of prisoners, or rather Jews, are required, to be supplied by the KL Auschwitz.*
- *June 1, 1943 Brandt called me with a request that I should assist him by placing prisoners at his disposal for research work into the cause of contagious jaundice (hepatitis) ... the work is being carried out up to now ... with the participation of the Robert Koch Institute ... in order to increase our knowledge ... of vaccination ... from men to animals the reverse way ... [and the] vaccination of the cultivated virus germ into humans. One must reckon on cases of death.*
- *Letter to Pohl May 1944: ... experiments with a view to producing a new kind of spotted fever serum ... 100 suitable prisoners to Natzweiler for this purpose.*
- *Brandt to Sievers March 29, 1942: ... sub-atmospheric pressure experiments ... on concentration inmates in the Dachau camp by the air force ... approved (by) ... Dr Rascher.*

- *Rascher to Himmler April 5, 1942: 'Highly esteemed Reich leader: enclosed is the interim report on the low-pressure experiments so far conducted in the concentration camp of Dachau. Only continuous experiments at altitudes higher than 10.5 kilometres resulted in death ... breathing stopped after about 30 minutes ... the heart continued for another 20 minutes ... after 4 minutes the experimental subject began to perspire and to wiggle his head, after 5 minutes cramps occurred, between 6 and 10 minutes breathing increased in speed and the experimental subject became unconscious ... breathing slowed down to three breaths a minute, finally stopping altogether. Severe cyanosis developed and foam appeared at the mouth.*

- *'One hour later after breathing had stopped, spinal marrow was completely severed and the brain was removed ... the action of the [heart] stopped for 40 seconds. It then renewed its action, coming to a complete standstill 8 minutes later. A heavy ... oedema [swelling] was found in the brain ... a considerable quantity of air was discovered.'*

- *Rascher to Himmler: '... principal experiments [concern] ... Jewish professional criminals who have committed race pollution ... embolism was investigated in 10 cases ... some subjects died during continuous high-altitude exposure ... some experimental subjects were kept under water until they died.'*

- *Rascher (concerning intense cooling experiments in Dachau) September 10, 1942: ... immersion in cold water in complete flying uniform ... with an aviator's helmet ... at water temperatures varying from 2.5 to 12oC ... large amounts of free blood ... found in the [skull].*

- *Holzloehner, Rascher and Finke reported on October 10, 1942 ... placed in water under narcosis ... certain arousing effect ... a few cases of excitation ... defensive movement ceased after about 5 minutes ... progressive rigor ... arms flexed and pressed to the body ... twitchings... ended fatally.*

- *Rascher to Brandt October 20, 1942: ['Warming with body heat.'] The Great Luftwaffe Conference on Freezing takes place on October 25. Reich Leader orders that the experiments on warming through body heat must absolutely be conducted [in time] … four gypsy women [to be] procured at once from another camp … have the low-pressure chamber ready for use.*

The aftermath

The principles derived from Nuremberg form the basis for later war crimes prosecutions. 'Informed consent' to experimental procedures is considered a paramount need, particularly when a doctor or other researcher introduces a novel experimental program.

In 2006 the *Al-Jazeera News Network* published shocking images of civilian bomb casualties in an Iraqi hospital. Many observers felt that the boundaries of decency and discretion had been transgressed by the needless and repeated exposure of gruesome footage — a complaint levelled against both the media and medical staff involved.

Twenty-five Japanese doctors were put on trial in Japan between 1946 and 1948 for improperly controlled experimentation on involuntary subjects. Seven were hanged, 16 were imprisoned for life and two received long prison sentences. Never before had Japanese doctors been convicted *en masse* for crimes that ran counter to the ethics of medicine although similar experiments had been conducted by the Japanese Germ Warfare Unit in northern China, which accounted for the deaths of 10,000 Chinese and Allied prisoners.

In 2006, Dr Akira Makino of the Imperial Japanese Navy Medical Corps admitted to conducting vivisections on 30 prisoners of war in the Philippines during WWII. He had carried out amputations, stitching of blood vessels and explorations of the abdominal cavity. At the end of his experiments, his 'patients' were strangled. It seems he had lectured high school students for years about his war experiences without once mentioning his real activities. As an act of atonement, Makino now desires to tell the truth to the world.

Remarkably, the US government is said to have secretly granted immunity from war crimes prosecution to some Japanese doctors involved in medical experiments because the US wished to monopolise the scientific data collected. In what was regarded as 'national interest and security', the government had thus engaged in what English common law would call 'complicity after the fact' — by covering-up horrifying Japanese medical crimes for six decades.

More recent aberrations

Much has been made of the violation of medical ethics in Abu Ghraib prison in Iraq, in Afghanistan and in Guantanamo Bay, Cuba. It is alleged that military doctors broke accepted rules of humanitarian law by divulging detainees' medical records to military interrogators in order to facilitate the extraction of information, or by failing to report prisoner abuse and by obfuscation or delay in writing death certificates.

While many of these alleged violations remain to be verified, it appears that some prisoners in Afghanistan and Iraq who died as a result of torture were medically labelled as having 'natural' deaths. In 1990 when the Armed Forces Institute of Pathology in Washington investigated autopsies of foreign soldiers and civilians who died while under the jurisdiction of US armed forces, some forensic evidence suggested medical collusion with the military.

All health professionals serving in the military are liable to find themselves in situations of 'dual loyalty'– caught between the obligation to help a person under their care medically and an expectation to act usefully to military forces. Civilians are similarly challenged. Some typical civilian and military examples are:

- Military doctors pressured to conceal medical evidence of torture when examining prisoners, as claimed in Mexico, Iraq, Afghanistan and Guantanamo Bay.
- Medical procedures serving the State rather than the patient such as lethal injections of prisoners on death row. Saddam Hussein habitually coerced his doctors into practising sterilisation and the amputation of limbs, genitals or ears.
- Practising racial discrimination against coloured people in the US and in South Africa. Many blacks in the US receive a lower quality of medical care than that available to others in the same circumstances. This may be seen as a more 'passive' form of discrimination by withholding certain tests and treatments. In South Africa, confirmed colour discrimination in medicine was once considered lawful.
- Remaining silent for military, legal, cultural or social reasons about a patient's health status and the reasons for it, such as failing to report certain injuries or to specify their causes or their relationship to death.

The American Psychological Association has directed its members not to become involved in any aspect of torture or other inhumane or degrading treatment, even if they choose to be 'consultants' in 'information-gathering' procedures. The US Department of Defense has also agreed that it is unacceptable to transfer prisoners to countries, such as Egypt, which allow their torture.

When 68 detainees' deaths — 'natural, criminal and justified [military] homicide' — were reviewed in 2004, the Pentagon claimed that there was no evidence that 'final' death certificates had been falsified by doctors, even when the considered cause of death had, over time, been changed from 'natural' to 'homicide', and vice versa. Reasonably, the authorities pointed out that without complete, expeditious autopsies in ideal circumstances, some initial interpretations could never be confirmed.

Similarly, the Armed Forces Institute of Pathology observed: '*When the cause of death is* [initially] *undetermined, the doctor will make a statement to that effect. When the cause of death is finally determined, a supplemental report will be made.*' Thus, in the case of a death which was still under investigation, the death certificate should indicate the cause as '*pending investigation*' rather than offering a misleading or hypothetical assumption.

Regardless of the obstacles to high-quality forensic medicine in the chaotic environment of war when autopsy facilities are usually inadequate and often far removed from prisons, the UN and the World Medical Association have agreed that, when examining any corpse, all doctors should actively seek evidence of torture such as *beatings, burns, fractures, pressure marks on the penis or limbs, torn ligaments, suffocation, widespread brain damage and uro-genital trauma.* All of these signs of gross abuse have been reported by doctors in army detention centres somewhere.

Chapter 9

'Disruptive doctors' and 'spurious peer review'

T he term 'disruptive doctor' is used to malign whistle-blowing doctors who criticise dangerous practices of colleagues or institutions. To be labelled 'disruptive' is not a benign charge. It signals but disguises an intention to get rid of a 'troublemaker' before any doctors or institutions can be shown to be guilty of serious misconduct.

The term 'spurious peer review' (SPR) describes the procedure which is employed to find a disruptive doctor guilty of misconduct, incompetence or other impropriety — whatever is enough to justify his denigration and/or dismissal. The essence of sham review is that its intention, if not conclusion, is known to administrations long before the review begins officially. Most egregious of all, the members of the supposed 'peer' group which may judge a doctor guilty of intolerable conduct often misrepresent their credentials and, therefore, legitimacy to judge the whistleblower's behaviour. Hospital administrations are wary of 'opening a can of worms' by allowing a whistleblower to go unchecked, even if professional destruction is the price to be paid.

That this fraudulent 'cabal' technique is extremely common in medical politics was reflected by a recent discussion of these topics in a distinguished US medical journal (*Medscape*). When a surgeon enquired about the definition of 'disruptive physician' — a term applied to him — nearly two thousand responses quickly poured in from practising doctors, all describing situations

73

where they, as whistleblowers, were maliciously victimised for acts of conscience and principle. Some of them were never again able to work in a hospital.

These are not matters which result in referral of a doctor to a licensing authority. The latter would not allow such arbitrary and capricious behaviour as hospitals practise behind closed doors. Since 'sham' (often called 'bad-faith') peer-review by hospitals was first recognised more than 20 years ago, it has grown to plague proportions, particularly in North America. It may also occur in job seeking and job retention, as well as in applications for grants and in qualifying for distinctions. The malfeasance is not confined to medicine, of course, but retrospective study of records is the usual tool of a hospital attack.

Inexplicably and unfortunately, courts are reluctant to interfere with decisions of hospital boards. Contracts may be broken without a reason existing. With accusers having immunity from defamation liability, 'peer-review' — meant to resolve hospital care problems in a fair and confidential manner — has become a weapon to indiscriminately damage the careers of targeted doctors by fake 'enquiries'. In its extreme form, the abuse includes well-publicised, summary suspension 'to preserve public safety'. That is a professional death sentence — an execution equivalent.

The usual sequence is:

- A 'disruptive' doctor expresses concern about safety issues or disturbs the financial comfort of rivals who may, for example, be billing improperly.
- Retaliatory claims are made against the doctor's competence and he may be suspended while complaints against him are investigated, rather than his original notification.
- Instead of a bona fide peer review of matters, a spurious ('sham') review is arranged with selected non-peers testifying without any examination of their claimed credentials.

- Summary dismissal usually follows and the original complainant loses reputation, job and security. Those whom he criticised originally are not investigated.

In the usual case of a spurious peer review enquiry held within a hospital, (unlike a murder trial, for example), the following are NOT mandatory: fair warning; immediate provision of particulars of complaint; presumption of innocence; exclusion of malice, politics and conspiracy; due process; proper procedure and rules of evidence; access to supportive witnesses; cross-examination of accusers; guaranteed 'peer' status of critics (their credentials may be falsified); legal representation; minutes of proceedings (they may be suppressed or 'lost'); reporting findings and reasons; investigation of doctor's original complaints and systemic institutional faults.

Lest it is assumed that 'only bad doctors get in trouble and it won't happen to me,' the following data are informative: most 'shammed' doctors have had no previous criticisms; 10,000 death-producing mistakes may occur in Australian hospitals yearly; one in every 5-10 Australian doctors reports a significant personal mishap to an indemnifier every year.

Presently, there is no professional body in Australia concerned, competent or substantial enough to provide expert, specialist support for doctors facing such a devastating life event as summary dismissal. (It is far worse than any medical negligence claim which can be professionally defended; sham review cannot.) Hospitals know that colleagues are disinclined to become involved — 'keep away from the trapped fly when the spider is feeding'.

Sham peer review has become a destructive tool for the use of threatened hospitals and doctors working in collusion. Substantial healthcare deficiencies must flow from the aberration of personal antagonisms and fears of exposure masquerading as good governance.

So who is a 'peer' and who cares?

The essential profile of a true medical 'peer' is quite simply (as the American College of Surgeons defined it) *being presently active in the same professional area as the doctor to be reviewed or investigated, and capable of performing the same procedures as those under review*. Obviously, there should be no hidden agenda or bias. Doctors who presume to judge other doctors' performance should first make their credentials precisely, freely and publicly available. That is not the same as hospitals insisting that they be published in enquiry records and they may be concealed permanently.

Until hospitals are required by law to adopt proper rules to strictly define who is qualified to be an 'expert-witness', as is already recognised by courts, this dangerous and dishonest aberration of justice will continue to conceal serious misconduct. Furthermore, the quality of patient care will be increasingly and permanently diminished by allowing institutions to conceal their own incompetence by expelling doctors and nurses who speak out about it.

In a unique and egregious example, a senior surgeon in NSW was submitted to investigation by supposed peers for alleged incompetence. An expert referee found no fault in his work. But his report was not immediately made available to those who employed the surgeon. The surgeon rejected a further offer of employment by his hospital and left its service. The Supreme Court found him innocent of any surgical fault but ruled that his 'expedient' contract allowed dismissal without given or even existing reason. Hence, he had no ground for appeal. Clearly, the intramural nature of the enquiry was unsatisfactory in every respect.

Jayant Patel's deceptions in Bundaberg were only discovered accidentally by an alert reporter. Most remarkably, it seems that, amongst the many statutory bodies concerned with the conduct of doctors, there is no statutory body presently authorised, obliged or bound to thoroughly verify the credentials of any doctor who seeks a hospital or other high appointment or who testifies in a 'peer' capacity.

Sydney ABC News of 17 July, 2010, reported that the new Australian Health Practitioners Regulation Agency (AHPRA or Medical Board of Australia) was set up to *register and accredit* health workers, as did the State Medical Boards which it is replacing. It scrutinises the credentials of those who are *applying* to be registered, particularly from a foreign country. The Health Care Complaints Commission does not have direct or automatic access to any doctor's CV, nor does the Clinical Excellence Commission or the Australian Medical Council, despite the last being concerned with, amongst other interests, education, assessment of international medical graduates, approaches to medical registration and the maintenance of standards. At this time, it appears that employers or legal teams interested in verifying doctors' claims of expertise are responsible for getting that information by whatever steps they care to exercise.

Chapter 10

Complex Australian cases

The following case histories have been selected because of their wide media coverage and their diversity. They detail matters freely available in official records and other sources included in this bibliography. Apart from the first case, no judgement by the author is implicit in their inclusion.

George Davidson, John Beveridge, Matthew Crawford and the Prince of Wales Hospital

These parties were involved in the 1986 impeachment of a senior cardiac surgeon. Davidson was greatly disturbed by the surgeon's repeated complaints of inadequate anaesthetic resources and hospital services for paediatric cardiac surgery. He often claimed that he could 'make or break' any surgeon by withdrawing anaesthetic services on the basis of his personal assessment of performance.

Beveridge was keen to recruit the surgeon, who was his friend and personal surgeon, to enhance his paediatric department. According to the sworn statement of A. C. Bowring, paediatric surgeon, he, Davidson, Beveridge and Crawford had met with the hospital CEO (W. G. Lawrence) in 1985, about a year before the surgeon's appointment to head paediatric surgery was formally gazetted by the Hospital Board. According to Bowring, Davidson advised the others that he would only provide anaesthetic services to the surgeon if Beveridge supported his early dismissal on grounds of incompetence. With that ultimatum accepted, but not conveyed to the surgeon, Beveridge immediately invited the surgeon to join his department to develop the surgical service.

On 17 December 1985, W. G. Lawrence, hospital CEO, advised that the Board of Directors had formally appointed the surgeon as 'Director of the Paediatric Cardiothoracic Surgical Unit'.

In May 1997, Beveridge wrote that he had no recollection of any such appointment ever being made to his department. Nonetheless, he had designed a door plaque carrying that title for the surgeon's office.

Six months after that appointment, and following 25 years as chief of cardiac surgery at the hospital, the surgeon was suspended because of violent criticism by a group of non-peers. Beveridge and Crawford led that group. They challenged his performance in such a way that his further employment in cardiac surgery was impossible and his reputation was destroyed. He terminated his employment at the Prince of Wales Hospital by rejecting any further appointment at that hospital.

Davidson never testified openly.

The surgeon had conducted all paediatric cardiac surgery during the preceding 25 years at the Prince Henry Hospital. Davidson had never given an anaesthetic for the surgeon. Beveridge and other paediatricians on his staff had never visited the cardiac operating room. Crawford, who became Davidson's protégé and temporary appointee to the surgeon's needs, gave his first anaesthetic for the surgeon in December 1985.

The surgeon was the only member of the hospital staff with a long-term, nationally and internationally-respected experience of children's heart surgery. That recognition was reflected in an expert, external, surgical referee nominated by the Royal Australasian College of Surgeons and the hospital to enquire into the surgical record.

Apart from the referee and the investigated surgeon, no other person involved in the enquiry had documented or significant expertise in children's cardiology, heart surgery or its management. The referee found no evidence to suggest that Beveridge was a cardiologist or that Crawford had recent, specialised experience in paediatric cardiac surgery and its intensive care, but Crawford was the centrepiece of what followed. He had recently returned from a fellowship at the prestigious US Mayo Clinic and was intent on succeeding in Davidson's service. Davidson, Beveridge, Bowring, the Director of Medical Administration and members of the Departments of Anaesthesia and Paediatrics advised the surgeon and later testified that Crawford had gained special expertise at the Mayo Clinic in the needs of the new cardiac surgical program.

According to sworn statements, the doctors, whose names head this case-history, initiated a private 'peer review' of the surgeon's performance between December 1985 and July 1986.

Beveridge and Crawford would collect evidence of any surgical difficulties which they perceived, with a view to suggest surgical incompetence.

With great enthusiasm to establish the new enterprise, the surgeon asked his friend, Beveridge, to expedite the appointment of experienced resident and operating staff and operating time and, vitally, the urgent appointment of an expert cardiologist. He was assured that Crawford had been highly trained in all aspects of childhood cardiac surgical care.

Beveridge begged for time to provide what was essential to make the new enterprise work. Meantime, he would share his own staff with the surgeon and 'work alongside him' in every respect.

That was not to be. Beveridge wished to dictate every aspect of perioperative patient care. He exercised his authority through his resident staff and through Crawford who had continued to claim substantial expertise in paediatric cardiac surgical care. Beveridge's intrusion into critical care in matters of which he had no significant experience created great administrative problems for the surgeon and risks for his patients. In effect, he had no continuity of control over outcomes and no personal staff to assist in his procedures.

Within the first early months of tedious surgical development, the surgeon found it necessary to live in the hospital in order to advise and participate directly in post-operative care. No amount of complaint by the surgeon changed Beveridge's authoritarian conduct. The situation was worsened by Crawford's obvious lack of significant experience and his domination by Beveridge.

The situation rapidly unravelled in early 1986. There had been no provision of the proper facilities the surgeon had demanded of Beveridge who refused to relinquish his invasion of patient care. Confronted by procedures of high complexity at that time, Crawford admitted that his personal, paediatric cardiac experience at the Mayo Clinic had been insignificant. He said his specific purpose there had been to learn about neurosurgical anaesthesia. A report from the Mayo Clinic showed his general rotation of duty contained no paediatric or cardiac component.

In June 1986, the surgeon advised the CEO, Lawrence, that he was no longer willing to proceed with the surgical program which was dangerously out of control and that his authority had been entirely usurped by Beveridge and Crawford. With no further discussion with the surgeon or apparent investigation into the surgeon's concerns, the hospital suddenly suspended him pending an enquiry into his surgical performance. About a month later, violently destructive reports from Crawford and Beveridge were served on the surgeon. Lesser criticisms came from others who had never been involved in the surgeon's work but who relied on Crawford's alleged expertise and his testimony.

What followed was a stereotyped, predetermined investigation ('sham peer review' as described in Chapter 9) into every aspect of the situation except the dangerous truth. Only the surgeon was examined or criticised. He was advised that he no longer had the support of Beveridge, Crawford or Bruce Currie (his surgical assistant). In fact, Currie stated that he had been coerced into collaboration with the enquiry and that he had witnessed no fault in the surgical cases which he understood.

Apart from the referee and the investigated surgeon, there was no expert present on the occasion of the surgeon's attendance. The referee had no voting role. Nonetheless, the enquiry was limited to an examination of severe surgical criticisms from 'peers' whose credentials had not been scrutinised and who were not peers by any recognised criteria.

The committee of enquiry exhibited no due process, minutes, procedural fairness, natural justice or legal representation for the surgeon. No hospital doctor was involved in the committee's judgement. The expected head of surgery stated he was there only as an observer. The expected head of medicine was not present, without explanation. After months of deliberation and statements from staff who had never been involved in cardiac surgery or observed it at the Prince of Wales Hospital, the expert referee reported favourably about the surgery but critically about its support services. He had provided a copy of his report to the surgeon. The committee of enquiry composed its advice to the board without waiting for the report. A few days later, Beveridge visited the surgeon's home unannounced, and described himself as 'Judas'.

The NSW Supreme Court, the Department of Health and the NSW Medical Board found no evidence of surgical incompetence. The court found that the surgeon's contract allowed his dismissal without a reason existing. Inexplicably, the court was not made aware of the insignificant cardiac content of Crawford's and Beveridge's CVs.

During the next ten years, the referee's report was repeatedly lost or mislaid by the hospital and the Department of Health. A frustrated Minister for Health (Dr Andrew Refshauge) finally sent his personal driver to obtain a copy of the report from the surgeon's home. He made no criticism of the surgeon's record.

Ten years later, Health Minister Craig Knowles made no criticism of the surgeon.

→

A detailed analysis by the surgeon of every aspect of this affair was published by Associate Professor Brian Martin in 1997. Copies were sent to 15 involved parties inviting their written submission of comments and corrections for simultaneous publication alongside the surgeon's report. Most offered no comment. Only Crawford and Beveridge responded in any detail to the surgeon's publication but both refused to write any rebuttal for publication. The essential facts of the matter as they are known to the surgeon remain unchanged.

Since then, copies of the surgeon's published story have also been made available to the hospital and the Department of Health, to Federal and State political leaders, to other health authorities and medical boards, to media leaders, Whistleblowers Australia and to many private parties who expressed interest. Although this appears to be a typical, highly destructive example of malicious 'sham peer review', it seems to be unique in Australia, especially against a specialist of unusual accomplishment. Surely there have been many similar cases which have been concealed or tolerated by submissive victims. *

Dr Aggrey Kiyingi, an Australia-based cardiologist, and two others were found not guilty of murdering Kiyingi's wife in Uganda. She had been killed by a hail of bullets as she returned home in July 2006 when her husband was in Sydney. Prosecutors said that the doctor had ordered the killing by phone from Sydney where he was in practice. One of the co-accused confessed to being the killer but died mysteriously in a Ugandan prison. The judge said that he was not prepared to rely on circumstantial evidence. The doctor was therefore discharged without conviction. He is still described as 'based in Sydney'. He

* The NSW Health Department has never acknowledged or denied any part of this case history.

is reported to have remarried in Kenya in December 2009 and to have discussed plans to build a large cardiac centre in Uganda.

Dr Allan Cala, a highly-reputed Australian forensic pathologist, determined that the cause of death of a couple discovered in their car in 2000 had been an accident. Additional evidence suggested that the couple's adopted son had drugged and smothered them. A year later, the case was reopened with a second pathologist's report. The adopted son was convicted and Dr Cala frankly admitted an original error. The HCCC disciplined the doctor who went to work in South Australia where the NSW proceedings were apparently not then thought prejudicial to his employment.

Dr Andrew Hollo is a well-regarded general practitioner in Sydney. In 2002 he gave an elderly patient an injection of Vitamin B12, apparently a common aspect of his prescribing practice. Later that day she collapsed with a stroke. Blood tests showed a potentially lethal level of insulin. Dr Hollo knew she was not a diabetic. As an advocate of euthanasia he was under suspicion, especially as the patient's will left him $128,000.00. Hollo was charged with poisoning with intent to murder. He initially said that he could not recall injecting the patient at all but in a later police interview he admitted giving her a Vitamin B12 injection. He denied administering insulin. He further admitted that his records were not 'up to scratch', he had been 'too casual' and 'the whole thing was an absolute muddle in my head'.

A magistrate dismissed the case against Hollo on the grounds of inconsistency in witnesses' statements and other problems in evidence when other parties were also under some degree of suspicion. The patient maintained Hollo's innocence before she died four months after he had been charged. He remained practising throughout the court hearings, and continues as a respected GP in Double Bay, Sydney.

Mohamed Haneef was a 27-year-old foreign graduate working in a Gold Coast hospital when he was arrested by

Australian Federal Police and Queensland Police at Brisbane Airport in 2007 as he was preparing to leave Australia on a one-way ticket to India. He and another foreign medical graduate were under suspicion of involvement in terrorist bomb attacks in Britain. Haneef was not an Australian citizen. He had trained in India and was recruited to Australia from Liverpool, England on a temporary visa.

The events surrounding Haneef's arrest on July 2, 2007 and detention for 25 days after claims of his involvement in the UK bombings are somewhat obscure and were the subject of a long investigation by the Australian Federal Police. It appears that he was interviewed on several occasions before his release on bail on July 16, 2007. Shortly after, his visa was cancelled.

Any case against him collapsed for want of evidence but claims of overreaction, victimisation, the possible concealment of interview records, improper arrest, detention and damage to professional reputation have attracted intense debate. Haneef's solicitors claimed that he was prejudged to be guilty by the Department of Immigration and Citizenship.

From India and the Middle East where Haneef has been since his release from custody, he maintains his complete innocence and expresses impatience to return to Australia to prove it. With a change of Federal Government since Haneef's arrest in July 2007, much has been made of the clumsy prior handling of his arrest and detention. He has, apparently, not been subjected to a medical board investigation.

While further information from the Australian Federal Police's investigations was awaited, it seemed unusual for a Federal Government to be simultaneously pursuing an independent legal enquiry which found no misconduct by Haneef. His experience emphasises the complexities confronting foreign graduates and the need for exhaustive enquiry before a suspicion of improper conduct is allowed to arise.

As far as is known, Haneef practises overseas and has not applied to return to Australia on his, allegedly, unaffected '457 temporary, long-stay visa'. In July 2010, he brought a defamation action against the Federal Minister responsible for his 2007 experiences and, in January 2011, the claim was settled out of court.

William Bland was born in 1789 in London and died in Sydney in 1868. As a British Royal Navy surgeon, he fought and killed another crew member in Bombay in a pistol duel in 1813. Bland was tried for murder in Bombay and found guilty. With mercy recommended, he was sentenced to transportation for seven years. He was imprisoned at Castle Hill in Sydney where he took care of other inmates. A year later, he was pardoned and began a private practice in Sydney. While involved in state administration he wrote a book defaming Governor Macquarie, for which he was sentenced to 12 months imprisonment at Parramatta and fined.

After returning to private medical practice in Sydney, Bland was involved in the establishment of a 'Benevolent Society' and the Sydney Dispensary. He became a patron of literary workers, built a church, developed educational facilities in the NSW colony, was involved in the establishment of a new 'Constitution' and founded the Australian Medical Association. He received little acknowledgement for any of these accomplishments.

When he died of pneumonia on 21 July, 1868, he was bankrupt and intestate. He was given a State funeral and buried in Haslem's Creek [now Rookwood] Cemetery where a large monument was erected to his memory.

Geoffrey Davis was originally trained as an anaesthetist but became more famous as an abortionist in the middle of the 20th century when abortion was unlawful in Australia. He had clinics in Potts Point and Arncliffe in Sydney and, as a matter of principle, worked with parenthood-planning, fertility and population services in developing countries in Southern Asia.

Long after abortion was legalised in Australia, Davis was brought before a medical tribunal in 1982, accused of failing to advise two women of the particular medical risks associated with abortion of late (3-6 months) pregnancies. The tribunal observed that Dr Davis had performed over 100,000 abortions in Sydney since 1974.

After much obstetric and gynaecologic evidence, Davis was cleared of negligence but warned about failures of his clinic to fully chart the post-operative progress of two patients, an undue reliance on verbal rather than written reports and disturbing inconsistencies and conflicts in his evidence. The tribunal was left with the *uncomfortable feeling that Dr Davis was at too-great pains to justify his conduct to a state of near perfection*.

When he died on October 3, 2008, he was acknowledged as a friend and saviour of thousands of Bengali women who had suffered during and after the military and civilian conflicts of the 1970s. He was accorded Bangladeshi honours at a well-attended ceremony at Rookwood Crematorium.

Reginald Stuart-Jones was a celebrated abortionist with clinics in Bondi and Rose Bay, Sydney. The author, Candace Sutton, wrote that *a knocked-up girl could stand on the corner of Macquarie and Hunter [streets] to be picked up and taken to a small private hospital in the East*. Stuart-Jones was said to have been distinguished as a playboy, nightclub owner, drinker, sly-grogger, associate of criminals, racetrack identity and an occasional user of firearms to emphasise his authority in the circles in which he mixed. He is not known to have suffered any significant penalties for these alleged activities. His death notice appeared in 1961.

Roman Hasil was allowed to practise in New South Wales despite a list of serious malpractice charges in New Zealand and a jail term in Singapore for domestic violence. According to Natasha Wallace of the *Sydney Morning Herald* (February 27, 2008), the NSW Medical Board had excused Hasil of serious misconduct in Lismore, NSW and earlier in Tasmania. He continued to be registered in NSW and Queensland as an obstetrics trainee in 2008 although it was reported that he had been dismissed from a Melbourne hospital in 2005 for alcohol offences.

Swapan Chowdhury was involved in female cosmetic surgery during 20 years of practice before a medical board declared him incompetent in 'basic skills, problem solving, patient management, interaction with patients and record keeping' in 2005. For some period thereafter, he was required to be mentored and supervised.

In 2007, according to Eamonn Duff's and Louise Hall's report in the *Sydney Morning Herald* of October 7, 2007, the NSW Medical Board again identified Chowdhury's substandard skills and ordered him to practise only under indefinite, close supervision. In June 2007 he chose to remove his name from the medical register after further disciplinary action was imposed. Nonetheless, it has been reported in the public media that he was later discovered to be working in four Sydney clinics. His current activities are unknown.

William McBride

In 1900, a German researcher had suggested that an injury to the nerve supply of an unborn child's limb might produce defects in its development. Because certain drugs could also block the embryonic development of limb nerves in animals, they might do the same in human babies. Fifty years later, other researchers found that a drug had blocked nerve impulses in frogs' limbs and damaged their growth.

McBride knew these pieces of past history and guessed that similar drugs to suppress the 'morning sickness' of early pregnancy might also damage limb nerves in an embryo and interrupt limb growth. In 1953, McBride was a tutor at Crown Street Women's Hospital in Sydney, preparing himself for consultant life in obstetrics and gynaecology. He was soon to make a remarkable discovery which changed his and the world's future in many ways.

Proof of that remained to be demonstrated but it seemed to McBride that about one in every five babies whose mothers had taken Thalidomide in early pregnancy for nausea and vomiting was born with stunted limbs. He supposed that all babies were not affected because of the genetic constitution of the foetus, how much Thalidomide had been taken, for how long and at what stage of pregnancy.

In December 1961 he wrote an urgent letter to the editor of *The Lancet* revealing his crucial observations of large numbers of limb defects in children of mothers who had taken Thalidomide for morning sickness. McBride recommended that women should avoid any unessential medication during the whole of pregnancy for fear of injuring a developing baby

Almost overnight, McBride became justifiably famous. He was envied and admired in an extraordinary flood of gratitude. Throughout Europe and Australia, in particular, he was praised, decorated and awarded prizes — enough to establish a research institute in Sydney called '*Foundation 41*' for further studies of the vulnerability of human pregnancy to environmental hazards.

Working with Dr P H Huang, McBride had also postulated that Thalidomide interacted with the DNA of primitive embryonic cells which were reproducing themselves at a rapid rate in early pregnancy. From that, they suggested that Thalidomide might inhibit the rate of growth of cancer cells — a thesis rated in the top ten of all Australian medical advances.

In 1980, he turned his attention to Debendox [also known as Bendectin], another anti-nausea drug produced by the US pharmaceutical giant, Merrell Dow. Perhaps unwisely, in retrospect, he appeared as an expert witness for US women who had children with birth defects and were suing that manufacturer. The drug was later removed from the market as a safety measure but there were many children worldwide whose terrible defects were suspected to be related to that drug.

Reasonably, Merrell Dow pointed out that, whereas more than 30 million women worldwide had taken Debendox, a minority gave birth to children with mal-developed limbs. Clearly, many other factors might have been responsible and nobody was able to say exactly which mother's child might be afflicted, even if Debendox was a suspect drug. Certainly, the lessons of Thalidomide could not be ignored.

The celebrated Australian author, Phillip Knightley, later recalled a comment made to McBride at about that time by Professor Jacques Miller, a distinguished Australian immunologist. After the astonishing plaudits generated by the Thalidomide exposure, Miller apparently predicted that many 'true' scientists, who spent their lives in laboratories without ever making a great discovery, might be resentful that a 'non-scientist', like McBride, could receive such adulation. They believed that he had just 'got lucky' with Thalidomide and did not deserve such publicity. By that time, McBride may have been too busy examining other drugs to take much heed of Miller's alleged warning.

In 1980, McBride's research assistants at *Foundation 41*, Phillip Vardy and Jill French, were conducting experiments on the effects on rabbit embryos of a much older, suspect drug, scopolamine, which was closely related to Debendox. In 1982, they were astonished to discover their names, with McBride's, posted as authors of a publication describing their work in *The Australian Journal of Biological Sciences*.

They were even more surprised to see that the results of their original experiments on embryonic animals had been altered, apparently by McBride, to show a much more definite and significant effect of the drug than they had demonstrated in their laboratory. When they anxiously confronted McBride about this, he failed to satisfy their questions.

Vardy and French resigned in protest and other staff of *Foundation 41* were soon retrenched. When they sent a letter of complaint to the Journal, it went unpublished. Under intense media scrutiny, the directors of *Foundation 41* arranged an independent enquiry chaired by a retired judge, Sir Harry Gibbs. He reported on McBride in the following terms in 1982:

It was moral blindness rather than error that led him on a course of calculated deception extending over a period of 5 to 6 months in his subsequent reporting of the experiment for publication ... McBride's misconduct in the period leading up to the publication ... can only be explained as emanating from a defect or flaw in his character. An essential quality of good character is honesty. Moral discipline is required for this quality to be held or maintained and it is given the name of conscience. His conduct in causing ... false and misleading statements and his denials ... of any wrongdoing, demonstrates that he lacked this necessary moral discipline to conduct himself honourably when honesty is at stake.

Already, the adverse comments and allegations of Vardy and French had been vigorously publicised by Dr Norman Swan of the Australian Broadcasting Corporation. The distinguished journal which published the apparently 'fudged' data also accused McBride of a lack of scientific integrity. He immediately resigned from all positions at *Foundation 41* but continued his consultant practice in obstetrics and gynaecology.

Understandably, McBride had been devastated by the accusations of scientific fraud, the enquiry which had found him guilty and the huge media concentration on his alleged misdemeanours. He was reported to have accused the NSW Health Department of being *a Gestapo state ... there is big money behind this ... big business is just as vicious as the CIA ... I have given evidence for the kids in America ... the drug companies have been known to resort to drastic methods to discredit those who appear in court against them.* Around that time there were rumours that some drug companies had, in fact, employed individuals experienced in intelligence work to investigate McBride's whole-of-life medical record.

To make matters even worse for him, he was then also accused by the Health Care Complaints Commission, under Merrilyn Walton who was not a medical doctor, of performing Caesarean operations more often than other obstetricians — suggesting that he did so for the sake of his convenience and income. McBride answered that charge by saying that his patients tended to be older, childless and more intent than average mothers on having a predictable date of delivery without protracted labour and possible damage to their babies.

It is not clear when the New South Wales Medical Board began its independent enquiries into McBride's conduct but a Medical Tribunal apparently spent four years in deliberation before its decision to penalise him was published in 1993. A member of the NSW Parliament suspected that the tribunal's performance suggested *a tendency towards government by tribunal.* An eminent journalist, Frank Devine, observed that it was the world's longest medical disciplinary proceeding: *The McBride case is a monster that grew beyond anyone's worst imagination, seeming at times to travel beyond medical and legal reality into satirical science fiction … justice delayed, is justice denied. The Boston strangler was dealt with more expeditiously and perhaps less expensively than Dr William McBride. What is the cost to date of the McBride Tribunal? Is there any limit on such tribunals? How much is each tribunal member being paid? I fear that this has developed into some kind of cottage industry. I understand that individual members of the tribunal are being paid as much as $800 a day.* Apparently, none of those questions was answered to Devine's satisfaction.

On 30/7/1993, after 180 sitting days with eight bound volumes of its proceedings, a NSW Medical Tribunal ruled that McBride's name should be removed from the medical register on the ground that he was *not of good character in the context of fitness to practise medicine.* There was a fierce polarisation of opinion inside and outside the medical profession between 'he deserved all he got' and 'he was victimised by the establishment' but he was professionally and personally disgraced. How he weathered the storms of humiliation is hard to imagine but, since that time, he has suffered devastating ill-health.

In 1994, the Court of Appeal rejected his application for reversal of the tribunal's findings of 1993 but he returned to work outside Australia. In December 1994, John Hatton, an independent member of the NSW Parliament, asked the Minister for Health many searching questions about who had paid what for what and to whom in the investigations and proceedings to which McBride had been exposed. As far as is freely known, no responses had been published within at least three years.

An application for review by a Medical Tribunal, April 29, 1996

The observations made by this second tribunal exemplify the thoroughness, precision, careful language and principles which such examinations observe. On this occasion, McBride was applying for restoration of his name to the register for the second time, having failed previously in a Court of Appeal. The tribunal concluded that his defect of character and dishonesty persisted. McBride had chosen to represent himself before this second tribunal and did not challenge any past findings.

The only question left for the 1996 tribunal to decide was whether, since 1993, he had, indeed, *retrieved his character.* He had hoped to demonstrate a resumption of habits of integrity, uprightness and responsibility and the tribunal recognised that was not an easy task for McBride. [His autobiography published in 1994 could have been to his disadvantage in his reflection there that he had not abandoned some of his earlier attitudes although he was claiming to have changed himself.]

The 1993 tribunal had reported on, *denials, evasions, attempted justifications and lies told in response to all questions.* It mentioned, *many opportunities for the practitioner to make an honest disclosure of what happened and to retrieve his good character. If this had been done, his conduct could now be excused. This did not happen.*

The second tribunal of 1996 was concerned about McBride's continuing lack of insight and was still not satisfied that he had come to accept the true nature of the character flaw which had been detected in 1993 — nor, therefore, had there been a reformation of that flaw. McBride's false statements, misreporting and invention of data were regarded as evidence of *moral turpitude.*

The majority of the tribunal [with one dissenter] found themselves: *unable to repose in Dr McBride their trust and confidence to be scrupulously honest and straightforward in the event that some conflict should in future arise between his duty to be honest and* [his] *self-interest* [concluding that] *public confidence in the integrity of the profession would be seriously undermined if he were to remain a member of the profession.*

He was said to have employed the mental attitude that *the end justifies the means* in so far as he had hoped to distort the true results of laboratory work. Twenty-one years after that research publication, he continued to believe that his conduct was in some ways justified: *The question was not and never was concerned with his beliefs about the dangers of certain drugs. Even if he was correct, that was not a justification for being fraudulent and inventing data that emphasised his belief.*

An additional factor which had influenced the 1993 tribunal was *an air of evasiveness.* The 1996 tribunal believed it had detected the same. It wondered if his answers were, *simply indicative of a mental rigidity, a lack of insight or that* [his conduct] *represents a degree of single-mindedness.*

Regardless of what the tribunal called *extremely supportive and thoughtful testimonials tendered by McBride, including a former Chief Justice's graceful mention of McBride's humility and dignity*, it was concerned to not confuse his reputation with his character. It became an issue of protecting the community rather than punishing the individual. Thus, the second tribunal found that he had not redeemed himself by the age of 68.

It seems that Medical Tribunals universally find that *a lack of contrition, remorse and apology, dishonesty, persisting attitudes of self-justification* are unacceptable to them. McBride had not appreciated the fundamental need to demonstrate those qualities rather than to make explanations and excuses for conduct. Nonetheless, the former Chief Justice [Sir Lawrence Street] repeated his perception that McBride had recovered and had *re-made himself with all due humility.*

This special evidence was finally accepted as fact and was influential in McBride's restoration to conditional registration in 1998. Significantly infirm and then aged 71, McBride gave an undertaking to no longer involve himself in medical research and to accept supervision by the NSW Medical Board. He had no wish to work again in NSW but planned to do so in American Samoa.

In his autobiography, *A Hack's Progress,* the distinguished Australian author, Phillip Knightley, wrote extensively about *The Thalidomide Scandal: where we went wrong.* He was concerned that the British media allowed governments to assert that these appallingly deformed children were not their responsibility. For Knightley, it was *a terrible failure of journalism* to find that, whereas catastrophic events on roads, in the air, in fires and other disasters are followed by searching public enquiries, the biggest-ever drug disaster of its kind was left to the devices of lawyers to determine compensation.

In 1968 and 1969, British families reached a settlement with the Thalidomide marketing company, *Distillers,* which gave them 40% of what they might have got if the children had won a negligence action in court. Beyond that, the parents were left to go cap-in-hand to charities. (That situation may have been remedied by further agitation in 2010.)

Knightley accepted that it was the combined assault on McBride's integrity by the laboratory assistants, Vardy and French, Dr Norman Swan of the ABC Science Show and Merrilyn Walton of the NSW Health Care Complaints Commission which destroyed McBride. Adding to other criticisms of McBride, Walton had questioned his justification for Caesarean operations on 38 mothers, an issue totally unrelated to Thalidomide. A Professor of Obstetrics at Queensland University believed that the clinical case against McBride was *a vicious persecution, ill-concealed, without substance and thoroughly reprehensible.* On the other hand, a paediatrician described McBride as *totally evil and without morals.*

In an eloquent summary of the McBride affair, Knightley wrote: *But there is a tide in the sea of human frailty and I believe that it will one day turn in McBride's favour. When it does, the names of Norman Swan and Merrilyn Walton will fade while the story of Dr William McBride — his triumph with Thalidomide and then his Calvary — will be read for many years to come.* 'Amen', many of us might say.

Winifred Childs

This senior Sydney psychiatrist, feminist and apparent socialist, criticised conventional psychiatry with its reliance on drugs and an assumption of the superior role of doctors over patients. In 1990, she was struck off the NSW Medical Register by a tribunal which found that she had shown *'gross disregard'* for a female patient by developing a personal relationship with her during therapy which included intimate contact.

In her practice as a psychoanalyst, Winifred Childs chose a *'very egalitarian relationship, not a power relationship'.* The essential difference between hers and traditional forms of therapy was that she encouraged an equality of patient and therapist. Perhaps as a result, she became progressively isolated from her mainstream colleagues until, in July 1985, four claims against Childs surfaced.

A disturbed female patient, who had consulted Childs once or twice weekly for three years, complained to the HCCC that, for a year after those consultations ceased, Childs had continued their long intimate affair. She also claimed that Childs had broken confidentiality. At a later Medical Tribunal hearing, it was claimed that Childs had another improper, personal relationship, with a doctor-patient [not Gluskie; see below] between 1986 and 1988.

The tribunal concluded that the complaints made against Childs had been verified. Although the record sheet of a Supreme Court of Appeal in September 1990 did not set out in detail what constituted '*professional misconduct*', it was noted that Childs' conduct attracted *the strong reprobation of her professional brethren of good repute and competence*. Childs rejected all suggestions of professional misconduct or impropriety. Having offered *friendship and then sex which was accepted, Childs then told the patient that she was using her in an experiment to explore her sexual preferences.*

With the patient being an alleged past victim of incest and still troubled by it and marital difficulties, Childs' conduct was said to have shown *a callous disregard for* [the patient's] *mental and emotional well-being.* Childs insisted that her medical duty to the patient had ended with the termination of their formal consulting arrangements. She further submitted that the earlier tribunal had failed to recognise that her alternative school of practice did not exclude *friendship* as a tool of therapy, or even insist on strict confidentiality.

A similar set of arguments surrounded Childs' continued relationship with a doctor after cessation of formal consultations. She took the view that a close and/or sexual relationship could continue quite properly once formal consultative arrangements had been terminated. A tribunal had questioned that view, emphasising that its responsibility was to protect the public from the effects of medical misconduct. The Appeal Court of September 1990 upheld the decisions of the tribunals that Childs should be removed from the Medical Register for at least three years.

Today, a person called 'Winifred Childs' appears in a business directory offering '*family and parenting services, marriage and family counsellors, medical specialists, psychiatrists, public welfare services*'. She appears to practise psychotherapy in Glebe and to have been involved in the training of a new generation of psychotherapists. All references to her were removed from the website of the Australian Association for Humanistic Psychotherapy at some time since the *Sydney Morning Herald* investigated her and Gluskie's relationship.

Clarence Gluskie

This popular and hitherto highly respected psychiatrist's name was struck off the Medical Register in 2001 over a sexual relationship with a female patient with whom he had adopted a *father role*. It was alleged that she was encouraged to regress to childhood and sit on his lap. He also allegedly explained that children were often attracted to their parents and that his resulting sexual arousal was therefore quite normal. The fact was, he suggested, that *genital stimulation releases chemicals in the brain that promote bonding between children and adults.*

Gluskie had been a psychiatrist in Sydney for 41 years until October 1999 when he voluntarily removed his name from the Medical Register and retired to the country. [**If a person has already ceased to be registered, he or she cannot be deregistered, but there may be an order that the offender** *not be re-registered.*]

Nineteen months later a Medical Tribunal heard allegations that he had been guilty of unsatisfactory professional conduct or professional misconduct, had demonstrated a lack of adequate skill, judgement or care in his practice and had been guilty of improper and unethical conduct between 1992 and 1995.

Gluskie had enjoyed considerable eminence in the community with an AO for his work with Rotary International of which he had been a governor, and as a foundation president of an organisation supporting children and young people. In 1989, Gluskie had edited a publication: *Hope for the Children — Child protection and Wiley Park Centre for Pre-School Children*. In 2002, he forfeited his AO. His name was later associated with a report of a 'Commission for Children and Young People, Amendment Bill, 2007'.

A Medical Tribunal of May 7, 2001 detailed certain aspects of Gluskie's actions with a female patient. He had:

1. Engaged in inappropriate physical contact during consultations, allowing her to sit on his lap while he held her hand, kissed her and touched her genitals.
2. Failed to maintain proper professional boundaries when he telephoned her, gave her gifts and disclosed personal information about himself.
3. Maintained a personal and sexual relationship with the patient.
4. Continued to treat the patient.
5. Insisted to her that their sexual and personal relationship be kept secret.
6. Refused the patient's request to refer her to another psychiatrist in 1994.
7. Referred her to Winifred Childs, a female therapist whom he knew to have been deregistered previously for sexual misconduct.
8. Commenced personal therapy with Childs in the same year.

Gluskie admitted a sexual relationship but little else. He did not appear at the tribunal's hearing in May 2001 and presented no evidence. Evidence from the female patient was not challenged by Gluskie's counsel who did not cross-examine her. The tribunal accepted the patient's testimony.

It seems that, in about 1991, she had repeatedly suffered from debilitating symptoms related to hepatitis C, her marriage was breaking up and she was devastated by fear of her illness. When she was looking for *a Christian psychiatrist* she found Gluskie. It was alleged that the professional relationship began while she was debilitated, had no regular employment, was in financial difficulties as a single parent and fearful that she would die early and leave her children unsupported. In her own words, she was *without health, career and husband ... vulnerable on every front.*

Quite soon, consultations with Gluskie had become twice weekly meetings. He confided to her that *the best psychiatry goes on in secret* and advised her to tell nobody that she was seeing him. She followed that advice with a high sense of guilt but found Gluskie comforting. She regarded his affection as fatherly. He promised to *love her back to life* from a state of depression and poor self-esteem.

At the same time, Gluskie seems to have maintained a sexual relationship with his wife and his secretary. The patient found that discomforting but accepted it. They discussed little else but how much they loved each other, had intercourse several times weekly and she grew increasingly reliant on Gluskie as a protection against her worst fears. She was terrified of losing him when he advised her that it was psychologically healthy to learn to lie. She reported that he had mentioned that other doctors might view the sexualisation of therapy as *draconian, obsessive and irrationally punitive.*

Nine months into the sexual relationship, she asked Gluskie to refer her to another doctor but he refused on the grounds that, without secrecy, they might both be in serious legal troubles because of the exposure of their intense relationship. Gluskie's attitude to the distraught woman seemed to have become ambivalent and perhaps disrespectful but, during this period, it seems that he was supporting her with between $100 and $300 per week.

Childs and Gluskie in liaison

In March 1995 Gluskie referred the patient (with her insistence) to the deregistered Childs because he regarded her as capable and trustworthy in maintaining confidentiality. He told the patient that Childs' deregistration had followed some *minor sexual misconduct*. He paid Childs' fees for seeing the patient twice weekly while Gluskie's sexual relationship with the patient continued. At the same time, it was reported that Gluskie also began having psychiatric therapy from Childs twice weekly because he trusted no other therapist in Sydney.

The combined effect of Gluskie's and Childs' management was to promote an even greater sense of entrapment and guilt in the woman who was increasingly dependent upon Gluskie financially. Both psychiatrists blamed the patient for the sexualisation of therapy but, in March 1996, Childs advised the patient that Gluskie's behaviour was so erratic and insensitive that she should not see him for six months. During that period they corresponded by mail which was transmitted by Childs.

By the end of 1996, the relationship between Gluskie and the patient had become bitter. The patient was counselled by both doctors not to make an insurance claim for her hepatitis C because doing so would reveal the extent of their long relationship and that Childs, while not registered, was treating both her and Gluskie. Eventually, the patient revealed the whole story to a lawyer and to her family. Gluskie offered her $20,000 in reparation for any damage he had caused her. She took new medical advice which persuaded her that she had been sexually abused.

In so far as the relationship had been a quasi-father-daughter one, it may have had potentially incestuous elements. In early

1999, six years after the relationship with Gluskie began, the patient complained to the HCCC. In October 1999, while these matters were being investigated, Gluskie took himself off the medical register. The tribunal found that Gluskie had exploited the patient at a time when she was: *at low ebb, in need of significant psychiatric help and vulnerable to the distortion of a therapeutic relationship into an exploitative one.*

By removing himself from the register and indicating that he had no intention of returning to medical practice, Gluskie had largely protected himself from further investigation by a tribunal. It did not expect that he would ever return to practice and he was ordered to pay the legal costs of his patient.

The tribunal had no power to discipline Childs because she, also, was no longer registered and had not reapplied for registration. Childs' involvement with Gluskie had not been made public until 2005 when she claimed to have been unaware of Gluskie's Tribunal proceedings in May 2001.

→

In 1986, a US survey of sex acts between psychiatrists and patients found that most psychiatrists who confessed to sexually exploiting patients said it was in the name of love or pleasure. Twenty percent of them claimed it was done to *enhance the patient's self-esteem.* Other more subjective explanations were *lapse of judgement, impulsivity, therapist enhancement* and *personal need.*

Some psychiatrists invented a diagnosis to explain why patients are sexually abused: *they have an illness which 'provokes' the therapist.* Others suggested that their misconduct had originated in their *unusually high level of sexuality* or their belief that *sex is a legitimate form of treatment.* Others felt that *true love for a patient should be allowed.*

Geoffrey Edelsten

Edelsten was struck off the NSW Medical Register in 1988 for at least 10 years for 'professional misconduct'. So he remains, apparently, after multiple attempts to become registered. Incidentally, he was jailed for a year in 1990 for hiring a notorious hit man to assault a former patient who was bothering him.

His 'official' current website is dated May 13, 2008 and had been copyrighted in 2007 by 'Prof. Geoffrey Edelsten and licensors'. It is divided broadly into aspects of his life and business categorised as home, history, academic career, facts and fallacies, philosophy, endorsements, guest appearances, press, collectibles and charitable works.

In 2001, while applying for re-registration, he admitted that he had lied to the Medical Tribunal in 1988 but had since reformed himself: *My character has changed; I am reformed. One can see a change in attitude that should give the tribunal confidence.* His application for re-registration was rejected. The tribunal was concerned that Edelsten still called himself Doctor or Professor and claimed the title of PhD from a US university which was described by counsel for the tribunal as *not* [providing] *a bona fide course of study.*

In November 2003, he again applied for registration, claiming to have recovered completely from the *defect of character* which had led to his de-registration. Again, his appeal was rejected on the grounds that the tribunal was not convinced of his reformation. A media article at that time reported that:

He drives an Alfa Romeo, not a pink Porsche. He thinks a brain tumour [which] *he had removed in 1995 had something to do with his criminality. His DNA-testing company which grossed more than $50,000 a year a few years ago is now idle, waiting for a Federal Government decision about privacy and consent issues. He has ... agreed to pay $40,000 to creditors instead of going bankrupt over his 'hundreds of thousands' of debts. He works and studies more than 17 hours a week administering* *medical centres in outer Melbourne, where he mentors overseas-trained doctors and doctors who had conditions attached to their registrations. In the last 10 years he has amassed academic qualifications including a law degree and Master's degrees in science, medicine, health sciences and business administration from Australian universities.*

In May, 2008, Edelsten's multiple academic claims, including a Doctorate in Philosophy from the Pacific Western University in Samoa came to the notice of the Health Care Complaints Commission. It observed that his use of the titles 'professor' and 'doctor' suggested that Edelsten was registered to practise medicine.

Questioned by the HCCC about his financial affairs, Edelsten agreed that he had not been fully frank in an earlier dealing with the tax office. He also admitted that he had only paid $2,500 of a $166,000 HCCC legal bill and had yet to pay a $10,000 fine levied on him in 1988.

Edelsten's website describes him as a medical entrepreneur who revolutionised general practice in Australia and championed bulk-billing. It claims that he made changes in pathology delivery and in medical deputising. He had been a rural doctor in three states until he returned to Sydney in 1971 to take up practice and had owned a football team franchise in 1985. It states that he was involved simultaneously in nine practices in NSW, spent six days a week operating and consulting until midnight while also operating a nightclub called 'Centrefold' which had a *penthouse private club where people clamoured to be invited.*

A NSW Medical Tribunal had removed Edelsten's name from the register on November 28, 1988 on grounds that he was *not of good character* and was *guilty of misconduct in a professional respect* in that he had [my abbreviations]:

1.   Sought assistance [from a criminal, Flannery] to intimidate a former patient.

2&3. Attempted to induce doctors [in his practices] to over-service their patients *and* to accept commissions for referring them to certain specialists.

4. Had fee-splitting arrangements with other doctors for referring patients for ultrasound tests.

5&6. Claimed reimbursements for laser therapy provided by a non-medically qualified person *and* allowed her to perform operations which required professional direction or skill.

7. Knowingly enabled a person who was not a registered practitioner to perform other forms of laser surgery which required professional discretionary skills.

For those misdemeanours, the tribunal ordered that his name be removed from the Register for periods ranging from two and ten years, that he be fined $10,000 and reprimanded. At that time [1988], Edelsten was able to move from NSW to Victoria, re-register and set up practice. He continued until interrupted by a *criminal* trial in 1990 on the first charge listed above and was sentenced to 12 months imprisonment. He promptly appealed unsuccessfully against that conviction.

His name was removed from the Victorian Register on September 4, 1992. The criminal trial judge noted that Edelsten had also conspired with police and criminals to give the hit-man, Flannery, an excuse for not appearing before a particular judge of the Supreme Court who might have been harsh on him.

Edelsten appealed to the Victorian Supreme Court against the decision of the Victorian Medical Board to deregister him but it and four later applications to the Victorian Medical Board for registration failed. An appeal to the Supreme Court of Victoria also failed.

The NSW Medical Tribunal of January 29, 2004

Here, various aspects of the accusations, appeals and tribunal findings between 1988 and 2001 were reviewed. Edelsten had submitted that he had *considered and reflected deeply upon the matters raised by the Health Care Complaints Commission and the findings of the tribunal ... I am regretful and repentant in respect of all the impugned conduct and have unreservedly expressed my contrition and remorse.*

Clearly, the tribunal took cognisance of Edelsten's involvement with *a professional stand-over man and murderer to intimidate by threats or violence a former patient.* In that, he had reflected the *gravest defects in character as well as misconduct* [which] *did not reflect a one-off fall from grace but demonstrated a variety of totally unacceptable acts which reflected a contemptuous disregard for accepted standards for medical professionals.*

The tribunal then confronted him with his use of the title 'doctor'. [His website in 2008 used the title 'Prof.' — presumably meaning Professor.] Edelsten explained that he used the title 'Professor' in academic correspondence only but he used the title 'Doctor' as a result of being awarded a PhD from the Pacific Western University in December 1995. There was evidence that, well before December 1995, he had styled himself 'Doctor' in both NSW and Victoria, even after deregistration in both States.

He agreed that the use of the term 'Doctor' was not only misleading but it had deceived the Pacific Western University which had accepted his inference or claim that he was a registered medical practitioner. The tribunal suggested that he had understood the *relatively diminished value of this doctorate degree and had done so since at least the year 2000.*

There were later references to a multiplicity of complex concealments, defaults and financial irregularities. He was reminded that he had given an unreliable account of serious issues to a tribunal in 2001 and he continued to exhibit such a lack of honesty and frankness that his application lacked any prospect of success. There was no tangible demonstration of reformation and his application was so un-meritorious as to border on the frivolous. In effect, he was wasting the tribunal's time.

Accordingly, the tribunal found as follows [abbreviated]:

1. He had demonstrated a lack of frankness and honesty;
2. He had not persuaded the tribunal that he had recovered in any way;
3. He had not rehabilitated himself and was therefore not entitled to be restored to the Register;
4. He had failed to pay the tribunal's, and other costs, of this application;
5. No further application for review would be entertained within four years.

Postscript: Clearly, Edelsten is a very talented practitioner. On July 1, 2004, the *The Daily Telegraph* reported that he regretted that he had not opted for a somewhat *less extroverted, intoxicating lifestyle.* He was living a *quiet and happier* existence managing medical centres and a DNA paternity-testing lab.

On November 25, 2009, it was reported by *The Daily Telegraph* that Edelsten would marry Brynne Gordon, 40 years his junior, on November 29 at a wedding for 500 guests. He claimed that he was at that time eligible to reapply for medical registration with assets 10 times as great as his debts.

In July, 2010, he announced the proposed $200 million sale of his GP mega-clinics.

Gerrit Reimers

Born in Belgium on April 30, 1964, Reimers came to Australia as a child and became an Australian citizen in 1981. He studied engineering for a year before transferring to the Faculty of Medicine at the University of Newcastle in 1984 from where he graduated in January 1989.

Following internship, he was a medical officer with the RAAF until mid-1992 while working part-time as a resident at the Nepean Hospital. He then took up a post as senior resident in trauma and anaesthetics at Westmead Hospital until he commenced formal training in anaesthetics in 1993. By the end of 1996 he had completed his specialist anaesthetic examinations but required a further year at Liverpool Hospital before he could be admitted to the Royal College of Anaesthetists of Australia in 1997.

In 1998, as a fully-fledged Fellow of that College, he commenced practice as a consultant with appointments at the Ryde, Hawkesbury and Hills Hospitals. On April 7, 2000, he was suspended from medical practice because of complaints about his behaviour during and after operations on January 24, 2000 at Hawkesbury District Hospital and on February 4, 2000 at Ryde Hospital.

Critical complaints

The Health Care Complaints Commission (HCCC) brought Reimers before a Medical Tribunal which ended on November 4, 2003. In that hearing, 12 complaints were considered. They included the following:

1. *Self-administration of drugs ... between 1996 and 2000;*
2. *Unsatisfactory professional conduct and/or professional misconduct;*
3. *Lack of adequate knowledge, skill, judgement and/or care; and/ or ...*
4. *Unethical or improper conduct relating to the practice of medicine.*

Particular complaints were that:

- On October 9, 1996 and November 25, 1996 at Hornsby Hospital where he was an anaesthetic trainee, he improperly disposed of an ampoule of pethidine and failed to employ conventional measures in a technical matter in anaesthesia.
- On January 24, 2000, as a consultant anaesthetist at Hawkesbury Hospital, he failed to complete anaesthetic records.

109

- On February 4, 2000, as a consultant at Ryde Hospital, his performance was considered unsatisfactory during an operation after which a patient died. His conduct included inappropriate procedures with narcotics and inadequate resuscitation of the patient at the end of a surgical procedure.

The incident of February 4, 2000 at Ryde Hospital

Whether or not a reader has knowledge of any aspect of medical practice, a transcript of evidence taken by a Medical Tribunal in November, 2003 is both graphic and highly disturbing. A few parts are included here in order to illustrate the drama of the situation by his multiple, irrational responses in a situation where Reimers was involved in a catastrophe.

Galatea Price was the senior nurse in the recovery room where a patient [SB] was taken following uneventful bowel surgery. The tribunal accepted Price's evidence about what occurred. For that reason, and because of its significance, the tribunal set out in detail much of her evidence-in-chief given over a period of about 45 minutes.

The nurse's testimony suggested a diagnosis of a severe psychological disorder in that Reimers refused to accept what was clearly evident — that his patient had become moribund but he didn't recognise or accept that and that he repeatedly rejected help to salvage the situation. He blamed his equipment and his assistants for interfering with his management.

'I don't need any help. Why would I need any help? You guys, you don't know what you are doing; leave her alone I'm all right. I don't need any help I just want her to breathe.' When he finally accepted that he did need urgent assistance, the patient was terminally ill.

He rejected a second monitor, saying: *'Take it back. There is no need for that'* and repeatedly asking, *'Why isn't she breathing?'* By then there was no heartbeat. The nurse observed that Reimers *'wasn't under stress. I was expecting him to be very stressed at that time. He didn't seem to understand the situation.'*

Only when a senior doctor had arrived to take over did Reimers begin to ventilate the patient's lungs adequately with oxygen. But the situation was obviously hopeless. Even so, it was testified that Reimers then *'went towards the drug cupboard and began writing something.'*

→

The Medical Tribunal took a great deal of evidence, including that of senior anaesthetists whose testimony was critical of Reimer's conduct in general and in particular. Not only was his anaesthetic performance at fault, they said, but there was also evidence of neglect of normal resuscitative measures. That neglect, so bizarre when taken in the whole context of complaints against him, suggested that he could well have been seriously affected by medication at the time of giving the anaesthetic.

Reimers admitted that he had used marijuana during his university days and had commenced illicit drugs in 1995 when he self-administered pethidine at home. He claimed to have then ceased drug use until September 1996 when he had taken pethidine and Fentanyl while working at Hornsby Hospital. He had continued to use a variety of self-administered medications by diverting drugs for the use of patients to himself. At one point in 1997, he admitted that he used drugs whenever he could get them — daily if they were available.

In August 1997, the NSW Medical Board referred him to an Impaired Registrants Panel for the management of his drug problem. It appears that he may have continued self-medication and may not have adhered to the rehabilitative program recommended by the board. Whatever the facts were, however, conditions imposed on his medical practice were lifted in February 1998 by which time he had resumed regular drug abuse without seeking help or telling anybody.

After the tragic events at Ryde Hospital, he was suspended from all medical practice by the tribunal in April 2000 and attended a recovery group, including consultation with a psychiatrist. He followed the recommended regime intermittently and partially for the next few years. He told a tribunal in November 2003 that he had not taken illicit drugs since March of 2000, following the catastrophic events of February 4, 2000.

The tribunal's findings: November 4, 2003

1. Reimers continued to have an impairment even if it was accepted that he had not taken narcotics since April 2000, but (the tribunal) was not confident that he had abandoned their use altogether.
2. Each of the complaints made against Reimers by the HCCC had been proved to the requisite standard.
3. He was guilty of professional misconduct.
4. His name should be removed from the register because of his misconduct, which included deficiencies of both character and skill. The tribunal detected no evidence of a reformation of his character.
5. Reimers was unlikely to ever again be regarded as a fit and proper person to practise medicine. Accordingly, the tribunal fixed a period of 10 years suspension to be reviewed in 2013.
6. Reimers should pay the costs of the HCCC.

Comment

It seems that Reimers had hidden his addiction to narcotics for at least eight years before he was deregistered. He admitted to the tribunal that he 'probably' used drugs on the night before the fatal events of February 4, 2000.

There was much media criticism of the NSW Health Department and the NSW Medical Board for allowing a doctor, known to have had an addiction problem in 1996, to return to full practice rights in 1998 — six months after rehabilitation began

— and be free to resume drug abuse from then until February 2000 when he last practised. [In 2001, he had been acquitted of the manslaughter of the patient who died at The Ryde hospital.]

There was also criticism of the medical indemnity provider, United Medical Protection, which supported Reimers legally and financially throughout the long enquiry terminating in the tribunal findings of November 2003. United Medical Protection claimed that it was concerned to *protect a possibly 'impaired' practitioner, rather than to conceal his problems in any way.*

Reimers' history was raised by Andrew Tink in the NSW Parliament on May 2, 2006. He referred to the fact that Reimers had confessed to the NSW Medical Board that he had used narcotic drugs on the night before the fateful operation and he had conceded that his judgement may still have been impaired during and after that operation. Tink complained that *evidence of Reimers' drug abuse in several hospitals was not given to police* during his criminal prosecution for manslaughter.

Tink further suggested that all documents held by the NSW Medical Board had not been included in the material produced on subpoena during his manslaughter trial. He believed that the NSW Coroner should act urgently to determine who was 'lying' — the HCCC or the Director of Public Prosecutions. No response or further information has been published.

In October 2007, a Heart Foundation Travel Grant report noted that a person named 'Gerrit Reimers' had been financed to attend a European Meeting on Vascular Biology and Medicine in Bristol, England.

Jean Eric Gassy

Because of its extremely complex character, this case is presented in considerable detail. Gassy migrated from Mauritius to Australia with his family in the late 1960s. According to presently available information, the following time-line summarises some relevant matters:

1980	Gassy registered as a medical practitioner in NSW.
Pre-1994	Practised as a specialist psychiatrist at the St George Hospital, Sydney, where he had been Acting Director at some time; unsubstantiated claims of assaults, moodiness, incompetence and being 'disruptive'.
1993	Dr Margaret Tobin was appointed to regenerate a neglected mental health service at St George Hospital.
1994	Tobin notified NSW Medical Board that Gassy should be investigated as an impaired doctor. Restricted practice conditions were ordered.
1995	Gassy elected to cease practice in order to avoid disciplinary and therapeutic conditions of the NSW Medical Board.
1997	A NSW Medical Tribunal suspended Gassy's licence for six months on grounds of contravention of earlier conditions of registration and uncertainty of his then psychiatric state and fitness to practise.
1997-2002	Gassy repeatedly sought treatment for AIDS (apparently without a confirmed diagnosis) and wrote a list of antagonistic doctors.
Oct 2002	Dr Tobin was shot dead in an elevator in Adelaide.
Sept 2004	Gassy was convicted of the killing, with a life sentence
Dec 2005	An appeal to a South Australian Court of Criminal Appeal was dismissed.
Aug 2007	He sought special leave to appeal to the Full Bench of the High Court.
May 2008	A retrial was ordered by majority decision of the High Court which failed to reverse the previous conviction.

➔

Events of 1994-1997

Described by Melissa Sweet as tough and often feared, disliked or resented [without] a sentimental bone in her body, Dr Margaret Tobin had been appointed to a position superior to Gassy at St George Hospital at some time before 1994. Such was her dissatisfaction with his conduct that she reported him to the NSW Medical Board in 1994. It was recommended that he should not be suspended but should consent to a number of conditions.

After several consultations with a psychiatrist who was acceptable to him, he discontinued that attendance — a breach of the conditions imposed upon him by the board. He failed to accept alternative psychiatric advice or attend appointments. In fact, Gassy chose to cease practice in 1995 but did not wish to be de-registered.

As early as 1994, one psychiatrist had considered Gassy to be suffering a categorical psychiatric syndrome — a major depressive disorder. On April 10, 1995, Gassy gave evidence to a committee of the board which found that, while he was competent to practise medicine with certain conditions, he was guilty of unsatisfactory conduct in that he had breached the conditions. Again, he failed to attend appointed psychiatrists and ignored the board's letters. For this, he was formally suspended for six months in 1997, without conditions.

Various psychiatric opinions were expressed about him. Some considered him delusional and unfit to practise but others doubted that. There was a general impression that he was fit to practise only under supervision and subject to monitoring. Gassy expressed distrust of some of the psychiatrists whose opinions varied but there was a general lack of confidence in Gassy's *capacity for insight and judgement.*

Words such as *eccentricity, significant anxiety, balance and judgement* abound in evidence placed before the tribunal. At the end of hearing disparate psychiatric opinions, it seems that

115

the tribunal had been placed in a quandary. Its members may have been unable to form a firm view of the true extent and nature of his impairment. At that time, it considered that he had been fit for some time to practise medicine but only under supervision.

Gassy had deliberately flouted the orders of those who had jurisdiction over him. The tribunal pointed out that *it is preposterous to suggest that a practitioner, as to whose competence there is doubt, should be allowed to refuse to attend a board nominee simply because that* [nominee] *doctor has not measured up to some unstated ... standards that the practitioner seeks to impose.* Gassy could not be *allowed a right of veto over the board's choice of* [supervising] *doctor.* Gassy then advised the tribunal that he had a *'change of heart* [as a result of] *his ... realisation that this* [was] *his last chance'.*

Events of 1997 — 2002

Exactly how Gassy occupied his time and whether or not he practised medicine in this period after suspension is unknown. The following is part of the published police 'case against him' in 2004. [Gassy disputed it and the High Court later granted him a retrial.]

Using false names, Gassy hired a car in Hurstville, Sydney, on or about October 10, 2002 and drove south. He booked into a motel at Balranald as a bearded, long-haired man. On the evening of October 13, 2002, he booked into a motel in Adelaide. At 11am on October 14, 2002, he was seen, with a beard and long hair, (according to Melissa Sweet), in the foyer of the office where Dr Tobin was then working as head of a mental health unit.

Four and a half hours later, a man of the same description was seen to enter an elevator with Dr Tobin and two other passengers. The latter two left the lift at level 7 while Dr Tobin continued to level 8 with the bearded passenger. When she left the elevator to walk to her office, she was shot dead.

On October 16, 2002, Gassy returned the car to where he hired it which was near where he lived, having covered 3,100 kilometres. Fifteen days after Dr Tobin's shooting, police discovered two pistols and ammunition at Gassy's home. The ammunition matched that used in the murder of Dr Tobin. [Gassy's solicitor denied that claim and objected to Gassy's being extradited to face an Adelaide Magistrate's Court when he needed treatment for AIDS, required heavy medication and also needed surgery for an un-named abnormality of his tongue.]

Trials

After an eleven-week trial involving more than 160 witnesses, a jury convicted Gassy of murder in September, 2004 and he was committed to imprisonment for life. On December 22, 2005, the Court of Criminal Appeal in South Australia dismissed his appeal on multiple grounds against his murder conviction. Two of his grounds were that he was not fairly represented legally and that directions given to the jury in September 2004 were not fair to him.

On August 9, 2007, Gassy represented himself in an application for special leave to appeal on nine grounds to the High Court. In May 2008, the Full Bench of the High Court ruled by a three-two majority to allow Gassy a retrial which did not reverse his original conviction.

The 2004 conviction

Perhaps for the first time ever in Australia, security men attended the Appeal courtroom where Gassy was found guilty. The NSW Medical Board apparently feared that, had he been acquitted of the crime, certain doctors may have been at risk of retaliation by an accused who was said to have a delusional disorder. After all, he had already compiled a list of six other doctors who, he believed, had been unjustifiably antagonistic to him. There is no doubt that the trial and the background to it had raised the level of anxiety among those who administer medical registration bodies.

One of the issues raised by Gassy's defence was the integrity of some 'peer review' processes [see chapter 9] — doctors passing judgement on the behaviour of other doctors. It is generally assumed [but challenged by Gassy] that those who make such crucial decisions are bona fide peer-equivalents of the accused doctor. But a fundamental and still disturbing question had been raised about the authority of those doctors who choose to act in judgement of a fellow doctor.

Some believed that the Gassy case could deter peer-review processes because of the difficulty of 'indefinitely' protecting a witness from an obsessed person. It was also agreed that it was essential for 'peers' to be undeniably qualified, competent and objective. There is no doubt that 'internal' [usually hospital] enquiries are much more vulnerable to criticism as 'stunts' than 'external' enquiries such as those of a standard Medical Board. The first frequently rely on pre-arranged witnesses in a cabal format designed to neutralise a colleague whom they fear or resent. Gassy may have seen himself as such a victim for being a 'disruptive' individual.

'Inside madness'

In Melissa Sweet's own summary of her celebrated book of this title, she frankly confesses to some of her reservations for the following sort of reasons:

1. Dr Tobin chose to convert from a clinical psychiatrist to a manager in order to make more impact on her profession. She was a tough, uncompromising, driven, judgemental administrator who was widely feared, disliked or resented. Why?
2. An intrusive biographer has too many opportunities for unbalanced reporting.

3. All doctors who give evidence against a colleague are liable to retaliation at some time — verbal, legal or physical.
4. Serious limitations were: her incomplete data; second-hand opinions of somebody she had never met [Dr Tobin]; many key players being unwilling to speak; being unable to interview Gassy or his family; her doubts about claims that Gassy had once assaulted a colleague.
5. Difficulty in understanding why the rhetoric of mental health reform has fallen so short of expectations and why it was so difficult to get appropriate help for Gassy.

Result of a poll of psychiatrists: Sweet conducted an anonymous 'key-pad' poll of more than 100 psychiatrists who were dining together socially. Allowing for the peculiar advantages and disadvantages of a situation like that, she gained the following impressions:

- 90% of them had experienced some sort of personal stigma.
- 90% had colleagues with a mental illness and they had done nothing to help them.
- 50% of those who took action saw a satisfactory early outcome.
- 75% believed that professional bodies rarely helped impaired psychiatrists.
- 60% believed that their colleagues could not be trusted to maintain confidentiality.
- 70% had suffered some sort of violence from patients or colleagues.

Sweet reports that some senior psychiatrists were concerned that the NSW Medical Board, though highly motivated and of great integrity, may not find it easy to respond completely and effectively to the problem of a psychiatrist [or other doctor] with possibly impaired mental health. One reason was that psychiatric opinions about psychiatrists were often obscure, confusing and conflicting. Even when scandalous situations are obvious, such matters are publicised but, at the end of long and complex enquiries, many issues often remain unresolved.

Melissa Sweet's conclusions

While observing that Dr Tobin was a *gutsy, complicated, driven woman ... often disliked and resented*, Melissa Sweet's elegant documentary shows that Gassy had at least one small but remarkable advantage over her. He chose not to practise after Dr Tobin reported him to the Medical Board. By so doing, and regardless of how he might have exploited them, he retained certain privileges that might otherwise have been denied him.

Such were the conflicting opinions and dense terminology submitted by some psychiatrists, the NSW Medical Tribunal chose to deregister Gassy for an arbitrary period of six months, possibly because of uncertainty about how his diagnosis might evolve. In the event, Gassy became 'invisible' until he was arrested for killing Dr Tobin five years later. It says something about the imprecision of much of modern psychiatry that the NSW Medical Tribunal may have been left with such a lack of diagnostic resolution that it had little alternative but to adopt a temporising measure.

As he did in the three years before the tribunal's deliberations, Gassy continued to decide what treatment he would have, by whom, for how long and of what nature. Out of that uncertainty, Gassy suddenly materialised in 2002 and was accused of killing an earlier tormentor. He was not convicted until 2004. In 2005 and 2007 he appealed against his murder conviction. On the second occasion, the Full Bench of the High Court, having allowed him the right to appeal, granted him a retrial. In effect, Gassy had regained the initiative for the moment. It remained to be seen how the High Court could negotiate the forensic and psychiatric thickets which obscured events of the previous 15 years. The appeal hearing on August 9, 2007 was unsuccessful for Gassy.

Interpreting Gassy's psychiatric status

In a far-reaching psychiatric review of the difficulties confronting registration and disciplinary bodies in matters such as this, Dr Michael Diamond raised difficult questions to some of which the author would respectfully offer the following comments.

- If a truly paranoid doctor chooses to neglect what the board considers is appropriate treatment, it becomes necessary to institute disciplinary measures. Here, that involved the Health Care Complaints Commission — a very effective but perhaps less formal step than referring such a difficult matter to a Medical Tribunal.

- Different psychiatrists are told different things by the same patient [as in all other forms of medical consultation]. When a psychiatrist tried to assist Gassy to find him a new area of work, Gassy ignored him because he did not agree that he was 'unwell', which was a breach of the conditions of his registration.

- A Professional Standards Committee meeting in April 1995 confronted considerable conflict in interpretation of Gassy's mental status. Although some psychiatrists believed that he demonstrated 'paranoia' and others thought he was merely 'deluded', his capacity to practice was not denied, so long as he remained under supervision.

- In effect, the Committee's report was more in Gassy's favour than previous interpretations of his condition. An odd question was posed, therefore: How could anybody decide that he was no longer going to practice when, in fact, the board had supported the idea that he return to practice, albeit with conditions?

- Dr Diamond observed that doctors may have *significant personality disorders that cause them to be viewed in their workplace as 'disruptive practitioners'*. But do they really have personality disorders or are they just different from others? Have they always gone about life with conflicting relationships? If they have *disordered personalities,* the next difficulty is to understand what that means in practical, daily terms and what to do about it in the short and long terms.

- Without presuming any particular insight into or support for Gassy's situation, it may be useful here to consider recent problems in Townsville Hospital where there has been prolonged infighting amongst medical staff. One doctor there who observed the situation apparently wrote: *What happened ... was a failure of management ... the situation could have been fixed in a short period of time. Closing the unit was totally unnecessary.* On the other hand, the Health Minister's office described: *dysfunctional inter-personal relationships between key staff.*

- It would come as a surprise if any or all of the individuals in Townsville could be deemed to have what Dr Diamond might consider a *personality disorder, impairment in their reality testing or a lack of credibility.* After all, whistle-blowers' organisations, for example, are largely populated by individuals who, with no suggestion of mental disorder, are vehemently adherent to belief systems concerning fairness, justice and honesty. It would seem quite unreasonable to regard them as having disordered personalities.

- The complexity of Gassy's case is emphasised by Diamond's further view that *the boundary ... between a paranoid demeanour and that of a delusional state is difficult to clarify. That aspect has to be addressed very carefully, very patiently and in great detail. To elicit symptoms supporting a diagnosis of delusional disorder in a patient who is himself a psychiatrist* [and] *well aware of the definitions and clinical examination techniques, can be impossible.* This was an admirably expressed observation.

- Unlike almost all other branches of medicine, the highest levels of psychiatric evaluation remain limited by a relative paucity of 'evidence-based' decision-making materials. Instead, it has to rely on conjecture, interpretation, experience, subjectivity and, perhaps most importantly, mature, experienced and balanced intuition. Even those may be poorly discriminating in forming opinions about some elements of Gassy's conduct. His later legal and medical involvements seem not to have assisted very much in understanding those vital issues.

Jayant Patel

The 1998 Year Book of the American College of Surgeons lists amongst its Fellows Jayant Patel, MD, MS, born in India, 1950. It goes on to say he trained at the MP Shah Medical College and obtained a Masters Degree in Surgery. In 1995, he was described as a Clinical Associate Professor in Oregon and on the active staff of the Kaiser Medical Centre and Legacy Emanuel Hospital and Health Center.

In 2008, countless millions of words later, he languished in a prison in Portland, Oregon, awaiting extradition to Australia [to which he had agreed] on 14 charges of medical misconduct including three of manslaughter and eight of fraud or attempted fraud. A US judge was highly critical of the protracted process of extradition procedures by the Australian government and had indicated that Patel could be released on bail if Australian authorities had not finalised extradition within a few weeks.

Patel's background

Patel emigrated to the US in 1977 and commenced practice in New York State. In 1984 he was suspended for negligence. In 1989 he became licensed in Oregon and was hired by the Kaiser Group where he was regarded as a *distinguished physician* in 1995. When he applied for a further medical licence in Washington State in 1996, he failed to disclose the 1984 disciplinary measures in New York.

In June 1988, Kaiser forbade Patel's performance of the most complex abdominal operations, a limitation which he apparently acknowledged at the time. In 2000, he was again charged with negligence in Oregon and resigned from Kaiser Group in 2001. What he did in the next few years is not clear but, by April 2005, he had been installed as an overseas-trained, general surgeon at Bundaberg Base Hospital in Queensland, Australia. Essentially, he was in charge of that specialty.

He did not disclose his previous licensing difficulties in his application papers, nor did those who hired him investigate his past record. Within a few months, complaints were being made about his conduct and, after two very busy years at Bundaberg, he resigned on March 31, 2005 after taking several months leave. On April 1, 2005, he was provided with a free, one-way airline ticket to the US where he remained until July 2008. Charges awaiting him in Australia included fraud, serious misconduct, manslaughter and negligence.

Political responses in Queensland

On November 30, 2005, the Queensland Premier, Peter Beattie, announced a five-month independent review of Queensland Health. It was found to be *the equal of any health system in Australia*. Beattie added that the Queensland Government had made *enormous and far-reaching improvements to the health system in only six months* — all since he had announced the review and an independent enquiry into issues involving Dr Jayant Patel.

On April 26, 2005, Beattie announced that Tony Morris QC would head an enquiry into several things: Dr Jayant Patel's record at Bundaberg, how hospital complaints are dealt with, how overseas-trained doctors are employed and how to make more doctors available for Queensland. He took the occasion to congratulate Morris and his two deputy commissioners as having great integrity and independence. They were certainly speedy in preparing an interim report by June 10, 2005, enabling the introduction of a Bill to Parliament.

Beattie, who has unashamedly termed himself a 'media tart', said the purpose of the Bill was *to keep Queenslanders safer from charlatans such as Patel* and to make it ... *easier to weed-out and punish frauds who pretend to be doctors, and doctors with blemished records who try to dupe authorities.* Contraventions of the new Bill's terms could lead to jail sentences of up to three years, *whether or not they actually harmed a patient.*

At that point, it had been recommended that Patel be charged either with murder or manslaughter of at least one patient. There were then 29 recommendations aimed at improving the function of Bundaberg Hospital and 12 recommendations concerning Queensland Health in general. Those measures would be managed by a new group of professionals who would lead the reform of Queensland Health. [There have been many alterations in details of charges since then.]

In September 2005, the three commissioners were disqualified after Morris's behaviour was found to be *aggressive, belittling and sarcastic* towards managers and other witnesses [presumably, rather than against Patel]. A new commission was to be established under the chairmanship of retired judge, Geoffrey Davies.

Other forthright responses

Just when a more orderly evaluation of Patel's performance was replacing feverish criticism, an *ABC Health Report* announced that a medical historian [and 'forensic psychiatrist'], Robert Kaplan, had suggested that Patel could be a *medical serial killer*. Kaplan likened Patel to two infamous medical poisoners, one being Harold Shipman, an English GP, who was accused of more than 250 deliberate killings for his own profit. [There has been no suggestion made elsewhere that Patel might have derived unusual financial benefit from his work or deliberately killed anybody.]

By that time, an opinion headed *Scandals in Medicine,* apparently written by Paul McNeill in July 2005, had concluded that Patel was *Australia's 'Doctor Death'.* It linked Patel to at least 87 problems amongst 1,202 patients he *treated* [not necessarily operated on] during two years at Bundaberg Hospital. It listed in a somewhat amateurish way various errors made by Patel and set out the history of Patel's previous disciplinary history and surgical cases from Oregon in 2000. Interestingly, Patel had been given glowing references by six colleagues in the US, despite earlier claims of his negligence.

Later responses

In April 2005, a *7.30 Report* on ABC TV included interviews with several patients who reported disturbing problems with their surgical treatment by Patel. Although there are some differences in the figures provided, it seems that he had performed many hundreds of surgical procedures during his two years at Bundaberg.

The ABC interviewer pointed out that one half of all medical officers in Queensland's public hospitals had been trained in another country. A representative of the Royal Australasian College of Surgeons said that the College had no record of Patel ever being referred to it for an assessment of his experience — which was an issue for Queensland Health to answer. [In effect, Patel had been appointed without proper screening.]

On May 28, 2005, *The Age* announced that the latest commission of enquiry would investigate the deaths of 87 of Patel's patients, 20 more than previously mentioned. That may have amounted to 10% of all patients on whom Patel had operated. But the hospital by then had written to 2,332 ex-patients advising them of concerns about Patel. How those patients were chosen or responded was not made clear but it suggests that Patel had not actually operated on a large number of them and that the great majority of his patients might not have complained.

It had been calculated that the population of Bundaberg had increased by 40% since 1999 while the number of beds at the Base Hospital had fallen by nearly 40%, indicating a very high demand for beds and staffing. At that time, an AMA chief stated that *surgeons are traded on the international market like precious resources and the exchange rate and annual salaries offered in places like regional Queensland won't buy you a whole lot.*

Although Toni Hoffman, a senior intensive care nurse, complained about Patel on many occasions, there was some suggestion that personality conflicts might have coloured her judgements. While that was never demonstrated, the view persisted and, perhaps as a result, the administrators of Queensland Health, the Bundaberg Area and Bundaberg Base Hospital failed to respond energetically to her complaints.

Certainly, there was a general appreciation that many of Patel's patients were very ill or elderly or both, carrying high risks with any form of surgical intervention. An audit of more than 200 of Patel's operations by a group of eminent surgeons suggested that he was not the reckless butcher he was made out to be in some earlier reports but that he clearly lacked many of the skills of a competent surgeon.

The civil libertarians had entered the fray in mid-2005 in response to which Dr Russell Stitz of the Royal Australasian College of Surgeons told the *7.30 Report* that [as far as murder charges against Patel were concerned], *I would like to know the evidence before making* [any] *recommendation. I don't believe at the moment we have enough evidence to make a statement of that kind.* Stitz added that, while those cases were being analysed in more detail, *we can't be sure where the deficiencies were. They are certainly not only deficiencies of care on Dr Patel's part.*

The end of the beginning

Patel was appointed to the Bundaberg Base Hospital in April 2003 as a general surgeon. He was soon to be regarded as the *director* of surgery although that transition was not formal. Within a few months, complaints had begun about his unprofessional manner, poor surgery and, perhaps, interference with medical records. Questions were asked in parliament and an energetic journalist provoked a flood of claims of misbehaviour before Patel departed for the US in March 2005 with his fare paid by the hospital.

In November 2006, a magistrate was asked to issue a warrant for Patel's arrest and to consider his extradition from Oregon. Two years later, the charges had been revised to manslaughter (three), grievous bodily harm (two), negligence (one) and fraud (eight). The political damage to Queensland's Labor Party was extreme. Beattie's leadership came under severe pressure. [He resigned to take an overseas post in 2007 and the State Health Minister was asked to resign.] Almost every level of supervision of Bundaberg Base Hospital was accused of incompetence or obfuscation. It was suggested that Patel's behaviour had been condoned in order to retain him as a surgeon in an area where it was extremely difficult to recruit any doctors.

Inquiries

An initial enquiry concerned itself with the administrative structure of the Queensland Health bureaucracy. A second *internal* enquiry at the Bundaberg Hospital targeted only about one-half the number of deaths attributed to Patel by other enquiries. At the same time, the state of Oregon in the US was re-investigating Patel for misleading information about his level of surgical activity in Australia.

Morris QC's enquiry was closed down in September 2005 after mention of *a health crisis — back flips, somersaults, and blame games.* In its place, the Davies enquiry began in September 2005 and made far-reaching findings concerning not only Patel's behaviour but also that of many senior bureaucrats in various Queensland Health authorities. By November 2005, a state chief health officer and several others had been charged with unsatisfactory professional conduct in dealing with complaints about Patel and severe disciplinary measures were recommended.

It was acknowledged by all that Patel's egregious sin was to conceal his past record when applying for the job at Bundaberg where a specialist surgeon was sorely needed. Underlying his story is the parallel one of standards of care provided by others at Bundaberg Hospital throughout Patel's term there. Obviously, inferior capability of support services could have compounded problems in his patient management but that has not been strongly proposed.

Observations on Davies' report

By the end of 2001, long before Patel's arrival, morale at Bundaberg Base Hospital had deteriorated and senior staff numbers continued to fall. Several overseas graduates, some on temporary registration and still requiring supervision, had been appointed to fill vacancies. A year later, the relationship between the hospital and its medical staff had worsened. Surgery was suspect and patients were at risk.

In August 2002, it was decided that a position of 'Director of Surgery' should be advertised in major Australian newspapers. Wrangling about that appointment led to criticism of hospital management as being *dictatorial, unresponsive, myopic and inflexible*. With no appointment, the position was re-advertised, seeking overseas candidates through recruitment agencies and foreign media. By that time, the hospital was short of at least two specialist surgeons. It was looking for an experienced general surgeon who could be registered in Queensland.

Patel expressed his interest. There was the usual exchange of documents, including many which testified to his skills and energy. He was offered a one-year contract although he had not revealed his past registration problems, nor had his application papers been properly checked by the hospital or the health department. It seems that details of Patel's deceptive curriculum vitae were obscured or ignored or set aside in the rush to have 'any' surgeon appointed to the post.

He was certainly regarded as the 'director' of surgery and that is how he functioned. Before long, he was actually offered a continuation of his contract as 'director'. Davies concluded that the conduct of the Acting Director of Medical Services, the Medical Board of the hospital and Queensland Health was unacceptable and/or negligent.

At the end of two years, Patel had seen some 1500 patients and, according to Davies, had had *an enormous* [good] *impact upon the quality of life of many more Queenslanders.* The hospital had accepted what was on offer and, as far as they were aware, or as far as the Health Department wanted to be aware, Patel was a satisfactory appointee. By then, there had been a large number of serious claims made against him in a relentless campaign by some staff members to have him exposed as incompetent.

It was generally agreed that Patel worked very hard and long hours but undertook surgery of maximum complexity, possibly with little experienced assistance. In some of those cases, he undoubtedly exceeded his experience and he was often loath to transfer patients to hospitals of higher expertise until it was too late. All of these matters were disturbing and required intensive investigation.

Davies found a spectrum of opinions which widely varied in their regard for Patel's surgery. Some of the accusations approached incredibility. One medical specialist denied Patel all access to his patients, which meant that they required transportation to another hospital to be cared for by some other surgeon. It came to light that Patel had taken leave between April and August 2004 — apparently without a formal replacement — only returning seven months before he left the hospital.

Describing Patel as *a prodigious worker* who *saw over 1,450 patients in the course of 1,824 admissions, operated on approximately 1,000 patients and conducted some 400 endoscopic procedures,* Davies calculated that more than 20 serious complaints had been made about Patel during his two year term at Bundaberg. Nonetheless, he was admired for training his junior staff, he was the first to make rounds in the wards every day and he never failed to attend after hours for advice or emergencies.

He was very conscious, as he knew management was also, that funding depended upon high throughput. The Director of Anaesthetics at the hospital considered Patel was a reasonably good surgeon with routine work. Others thought him charming, confident and a powerful personality. Those were qualities accorded him by referees in September 2003 when an academic position at the University of Queensland was advertised and Patel won the appointment ahead of a Dr de Lacey who later testified strongly against Patel.

Denouement

From the middle of 2003, Ms Hoffman was a courageous, prolific and methodical critic who expressed her anxieties wherever she believed they would be received, despite sensing a reluctance of those in authority to want to know of her apprehensions. Her complaints included complications and deaths, Patel's personal behaviour, a lack of support for her from hospital administration and Patel's resistance to all criticism.

Others thought that he was old-fashioned, pessimistic about improving overall performance, too aggressive in his choices of operations and late to transfer patients who needed additional facilities. In summary, therefore, there was distrust of Patel's capabilities and his apparent lack of recognition of his limitations. Some efforts were made to limit the range of operations he performed but it appeared that he did not take that seriously.

Regardless of that atmosphere, being caught between having Dr Patel and having no surgeon at all, the hospital then offered him a three months locum from February 2005 while it looked for a replacement surgeon before he departed as planned. When he rejected that, he was invited to extend his contract for a further four years from early 2005. He rejected that proposal also and resigned while criticisms continued behind his back.

When a senior health executive finally visited the hospital in mid-February 2005 to evaluate these festering problems, Ms Hoffman felt she had been ignored. After she approached parliamentarians to raise her serious questions with the Minister of Health, something began to happen. There was clear recognition at all levels of administration that Patel's performance needed close investigation but, by then, he had resigned and returned to the US on a free ticket from the hospital.

Issues of procedural fairness and natural justice were irrelevant while Patel was back in the US but a protracted and detailed review process was initiated into his record at Bundaberg. All the while, the *Courier-Mail* and other media used the title 'Dr Death' for Patel and relentlessly promoted widespread resentment in the community at large about the lack of proper screening of him and the many lost opportunities to halt or place restrictions on his work.

An example of peer review

Some experienced surgeons who considered some of Patel's operations found against him. One was Dr Geoffrey de Lacey who had previously run second to Dr Patel in seeking an academic appointment. Inevitably, his criticisms might have been challenged for that reason. Dr Peter Woodruff, a former Vice-President of the Royal Australasian College of Surgeons, focused on patients who had died or had important complications or were transferred to another institution, amongst 1,450 patients seen by Patel during his time at Bundaberg.

His overall conclusion was that there were 48 patients where Dr Patel had or may have contributed to an adverse outcome. While he was very critical of some of his treatment, he emphasised that Patel's involvement was, in many cases, *incidental* because many of those patients were already mortally threatened or had terminal pathology. He also deprecated the possibility that there had been tampering with case notes by Patel. Nonetheless, he regarded Patel as an intelligent and industrious man who, in a different environment, had a potential to be a *productive contributor*.

Davies' conclusions

The Commissioner acknowledged the widespread systemic deficiencies within Bundaberg Hospital before, during and [as must be inevitable] after Patel's appointment. He praised Ms Hoffman for her persistence in finally securing attention for her apprehensions about Patel. He found that Patel had performed badly and dishonestly in several respects. He was highly critical of senior management and recommended that, in certain areas, further disciplinary measures were applicable.

Patel's fate depended largely upon his responses to each complaint made against him with independent, expert, surgical and legal opinions available to him. How he responded to these various aspects when properly represented in a court of law remained to be seen. He volunteered to be extradited to Australia on June 26, 2008, and had a legal team to assist him although he remained in custody until bail was granted on July 21, 2008.

Trial and sentencing

He began trial in Brisbane on March 22, 2010 and proceeded with full public scrutiny and reporting. After 59 days of court hearings and seven days of jury consideration, Patel was convicted on three counts of manslaughter and one of grievous bodily harm. A gaol sentence of seven years was imposed on July 1, 2010. It seemed certain that he would appeal that sentence on several complex procedural grounds.

Sarah Elks of *The Australian* reported on June 30, 2010 that such an appeal could well expose a legal minefield never before encountered in Australian medical history. His proposed appeal against all charges was confirmed on July 15, 2010. A week later, the Queensland Attorney-General filed papers seeking an increase in Patel's sentence. On September 21, 2010, it was reported that Patel could no longer afford an appeal; however, an appeal in early 2011 has now failed. Time will tell what happens next.

→

Patel's falsifications and misrepresentations are grave matters but certainly not unknown elsewhere in Australia. To label him *Dr Death* long before accusations and responses are known generated extraordinary, progressive damage to him. From that alone, and despite every possible legal precaution, his chances of a completely fair trial in Australia would always have been limited.

It is generally accepted that Queensland Health, Bundaberg Hospital bureaucracy, Beattie's government and many others are vulnerable to severe criticism for failure to discover Patel's deceptions or performance record before his Bundaberg appointment. Especially disturbing is the realisation that he was essential to the hospital's surgical functioning, a matter of profound political concern. Most remarkable is that he was paid to return home to Oregon after his refusal of a substantial offer of further employment as a senior surgeon. Curiously, there has been no mention yet of any legal firm offering to promote a *class action* on behalf of his patients.

Whatever else, the 'Dr Death of Bundaberg' affair has exposed high levels of possibly premature judgement by the community and of incompetence in the Queensland health administration. Perhaps some accusers may become less enthusiastic about further, more detailed inquisitions into Patel's history as time passes.

In 2007, I attempted to contact Tony Morris QC, Ms Toni Hoffman and Hedley Thomas [a journalist who led the media charge against Patel] about Patel's situation. None responded to repeated requests.

John Bannister

Bannister graduated in medicine from the University of Sydney in 1965 and pursued an orthopaedic surgical career. He gained Fellowship of the Royal College of Surgeons (Edinburgh) in 1972 and commenced private practice in 1975. So he continued until his name was removed from the medical register in 1992. An avowed Christian, Bannister had, by his own word, been preoccupied with creating the best and largest orthopaedic practice in Sydney.

It was said that he performed three or four spinal operations a week and, at one time or another, employed 40 secretaries to service a large referral practice, particularly involving workers' and motor traffic injury compensation patients, at his offices in Macquarie Street Sydney, Blacktown, Marrickville, Leichhardt, Fairfield and Wollongong.

In addition to practising as an orthopaedic surgeon, Bannister had been a real estate trader for some years prior to 1992. Before his deregistration, he had defaulted in mortgage payments with his liabilities greatly exceeding his assets.

A 1992 Medical Tribunal ordered that his name be removed from the medical register in NSW for several reasons:

1. He neglected to arrange proper substitute care and records when he took leave shortly after complications became apparent in two surgical patients.

2. He failed to keep proper records of the operations and his post-operative attendances. He billed one patient for ten post-operative visits which he did not, in fact, make — five of them after he had departed on leave.

3. He overcharged, or charged for attendances on, patients when he was *aware that he had not visited the patients on those dates.* This was regarded as fraud resulting from a defective billing system which he had devised

4. He alleged that another doctor had attended patients in his place when he had no confirmation of those billings. These matters of *deliberate deceit* continued for five years, reflecting a *marked degree of moral turpitude*. Bannister had been *caught out in his longstanding practice of charging for 'phantom visits'*.

⤍

A remarkable procession of attempts by Bannister to regain registration followed. Apart from the Medical Tribunal finding of April 1992, followed by an appeal for a stay of proceedings, there were further tribunal hearings in 1995, 1996 and 1999 — all rejecting his suitability for re-registration on the basis of lack of contrition, remorse, reform or change of his character.

In 1995, a tribunal also considered his bankruptcy and arrangements for payment of outstanding debts. It took into account issues such as trust, confidence, confidentiality and right-conduct in a doctor — emphasising that the onus of proof in such enquiries rests on the deregistered party to show that he had become *a fit and proper person to be registered*.

Bannister did not convince the tribunal that he accepted that he had acted *fraudulently, recklessly or carelessly* in his accounting. Moreover, he had failed to repay debts or otherwise settle matters to do with his bankruptcy. The tribunal observed that *since the previous tribunal's decision on 29 April 1992, Mr Bannister has made no reparations at all (up to 1995).*

There was additional criticism of his prescribing drugs of addiction without authority. In one case, he had ordered a restricted drug 115 times to one patient within 13 months and 57 times to another within eight months. Bannister did not agree that he had been reckless in those prescriptions although the tribunal had regarded his attitude as being marked by *arrogance, a lack of concern and a blatant disregard for the law.*

136

Finally the tribunal expressed grave reservations about Bannister's credibility, finding him evasive, blaming others for his own shortcomings and disregarding his obligations to repay his overcharges. The tribunal rejected his claim that he was a reformed individual. His deregistration was maintained for at least a further two years and he was severely censured for his prescriptions of addictive drugs.

Following his seeking leave to appeal in the High Court, which was rejected, he sought registration at another Medical Tribunal on October 8, 2003. He claimed that he had *overcome the defects of character* which had caused him to be deregistered in the first place. The tribunal was not impressed by Bannister's suggestion that reading out-dated orthopaedic text books in the Mitchell Library comprised continuing medical education preparatory to returning to practise.

It also noted that he had apparently corresponded evasively with an overseas employer in regard to the reasons for his deregistration and had continued to describe himself as 'a surgeon' or 'doctor' since deregistration and had misrepresented his surgical college affiliation.

At the end of a further rigorous examination of Bannister's attitude and conduct, the tribunal was not persuaded that the defects in character found in 1992 had been sufficiently overcome to allow him reinstatement in the medical register. *Greed, not need, was his motivator* in his fraudulent behaviour and the tribunal could not detect *a marked reversal in the traits of character previously demonstrated. He has an insuperable difficulty in this endeavour if he is unable to persuade this tribunal that he has been frank.* It appears that he has not been re-registered.

Eric Hedberg

Hedberg was an accomplished anatomist and surgeon who developed a large consultant practice in Sydney after WWII and was an esteemed member of the surgical staff of Sydney

Hospital. Neither he nor anybody else was ever charged with any misdemeanour related to this history.

James Yeates was also a distinguished surgeon working at Sydney Hospital — a hero of WWII in which he earned decorations for his surgery in the Middle East and the South Pacific. He, also, had returned to civilian practice with a high reputation, specialising in diseases of the breast. He was married to Diana and had two children at the time he was found dead in his garage late one night.

Following Yeates' violent death in September 1960, Hedberg was a conspicuous figure because of a suspected affair with Yeates' wife, Diana — just as he had come under suspicion five months earlier when his first wife had died in strange circumstances. On both scores, no charges were ever laid.

Hedberg had an unusual reputation. He had been mentioned favourably in despatches during his service in WWII. Amongst those with whom he worked, many considered him brilliant. The personalities of Yeates and Hedberg were apparently very different. Hedberg was 47, a few years younger than Yeates at the time of Yeates' death.

It was apparently common knowledge that Hedberg, who worked and socialised closely with Yeates and his family, admired Diana Yeates. Inevitably, both she and Hedberg were suspected of complicity in the death of her husband when the police and the media were confronted by circumstantial evidence concerning her and Hedberg. In no way does the writer suggest any such complicity. Nearly 50 years later, there remains a degree of polarisation of opinion about the matter within the medical community of Sydney at large and others who were aware of the intriguing investigation.

Hedberg married Yeates' widow, Diana, in May 1964 and they lived together until Hedberg's death in 2001. Candace Sutton has rekindled interest and conjecture with her remarkably detailed account of the matter in her book '*The Needle in the Heart*

Murder'. A great deal of what follows is based on her account of the matter. Some of the files pertaining to the inquest into Yeates' death were said to have disappeared soon after the verdict and have never been found. The following is what Sutton has reported:

Towards midnight on September 14, 1960, Yeates returned home to Vaucluse after a late meeting at Sydney Hospital. He parked his car in the driveway, walked through an annexe to enter the garage in order to open the roller door. His car's headlights were left on, its motor was running and the driver's door was open, apparently preparatory to his driving into the garage. By that hour, Diana Yeates and her children had watched TV after dinner at home and gone to bed.

When nothing had changed in the driveway for about five hours, wakeful neighbours became concerned. Near 5 a.m., one of them phoned the Yeates residence and spoke to Diana who phoned her brother. The neighbour and Diana met in the darkened garage and discovered Yeates dead on the floor with a large head injury. A broken light bulb was nearby. The police were called at around 5.30 a.m. Diana Hedberg sought legal advice within an hour or so.

By 8 a.m., her brother and a general practitioner friend, Dr Douglas Fearon, had arrived at the house. She told police she knew of nobody who would have wanted to kill her husband. There was a suggestion made by her brother and by Dr Fearon that Yeates may have been electrocuted by the broken lamp and had injured his head as he fell. The police discovered ampoules of adrenaline and a few surgical instruments in the glove box of the car.

There was no evidence of a robbery and there was no weapon discovered but there was evidence that Yeates body had been moved across the floor of the garage. The police found no evidence to suggest his head injury had been caused by a fall. They also found blood spots on his shirt near a puncture wound on his left breast. They soon wondered if Yeates may have been given a cardiac injection of adrenaline as a stimulant for resuscitation. Nobody admitted to having done so.

At around 3.30 p.m. on that day, the police returned to Vaucluse to interview Diana Yeates again. At that time, her brother was present as well as Dr Alan McGuinness, a Sydney Hospital specialist and family friend. He was the first of some 200 doctors whom the police interviewed in regard to the death. By then, Diana and her advisers had agreed that a barrister friend, Victor Maxwell, should be brought into the picture. He was the executor and trustee of James Yeates' estate.

Initially, police pathologists found it difficult to decide whether the skull fracture on the top of Yeates' head or a possible adrenaline injection into his heart was the primary cause of death. No stranger or strange car had been seen in the vicinity of Yeates' home on the night of his death but there was later evidence that Hedberg frequently visited the Yeates' home and socialised with all members of the family. On occasions, it appears that only he and Diana Yeates were present.

The amount of adrenaline in Yeates' body was extremely high. The question was *who gave the injection, why, when and why so much?* The police pathologists concluded that Yeates' head wound was not inflicted by falling and it had occurred at least an hour before he died. There was some doubt about the effects of a large injection of adrenaline into Yeates' heart but it was conceded that the amount could have been fatal.

It seemed quite remarkable to police that, four days after Yeates' death and having already given them a statement, Hedberg re-approached them to report that he had lost some ampoules of concentrated adrenaline from his car in the previous week. He told them: *I know this sounds fantastic, but as I seem to be the logical suspect, I have been wondering whether somebody has tried to have a shot at me. Knowing my close link with the Yeates' family, someone may have conceived the idea of using adrenaline from my car on Dr Yeates, believing that I would be connected with the crime and therefore destroy me professionally. I obtained the phials from Gourlay's chemist shop in King Street for use in the treatment of my youngest son, Peter.* [He said that Peter was an asthmatic.]

The police were very interested in this revelation. Hedberg went on to say that he had left the adrenaline on the front seat of his car which was not locked. He claimed to have found the ampoules missing three days after Yeates' death. He told them: '*It seems funny, doesn't it? You sometimes find that the person who sets out to help the police finally ends up being charged.*' He also said that, as a medical referee for insurance companies, one of his medical reports might have provoked the ill-disposition toward him of somebody on whom he had reported. He then observed that '*the most bizarre feature is the intra-cardiac injection given either to focus suspicion on medical people or as an act of vengeance.*'

When nobody at Gourlay's pharmacy could recall the sale of adrenaline to anybody in any way resembling Hedberg, the police concluded that they had a major suspect — reinforced by the fact that the family and friends of Hedberg's first wife wished to speak to the police about what they saw as an affair, a poem written by Hedberg to Diana Yeates. Perhaps as a result, Hedberg's first wife had revised her will to leave him nothing. Soon after, a domestic worker for the Yeates' family reported finding an axe somewhere.

It appears that Hedberg had diagnosed breast cancer in his first wife in 1958. She believed that he was infatuated with Diana Yeates and confronted him. Soon after, Hedberg's wife began to have fainting attacks, which he treated by injections after which she became ill. She apparently died rather suddenly and was cremated at Easter, two days after her death. Hedberg had apparently told family members that he had injected his wife's varicose veins with a conventional medication. He was surprised to discover that she had left him nothing in her will.

By that time, all concerned parties had taken senior legal advice. Again, the police raised the question of whether Hedberg had bought adrenaline at Gourlay's pharmacy. Again, nobody remembered him. Police repeatedly interviewed him and Diana Yeates. Both insisted on solicitors being present at all times.

On December 7, 1960, a Coroner's inquest commenced at the Central Police Court where all parties had highly regarded legal teams. There was intense questioning of many witnesses about the events surrounding Yeates' death. Diana Yeates and Hedberg sat apart and apparently did not communicate. Much was made of the 'poem' written by Hedberg to Diana Yeates on February 5, 1959, generally interpreted as an expression of frustrated infatuation.

The Coroner repeatedly made it clear that he believed that Yeates had been murdered and there was an impression given to some that he may have over-emphasised the fact that the police had been unable to obtain enough evidence to charge anybody. The inquest deteriorated into a protracted, bitter conflict between the Coroner and senior legal counsel acting for Hedberg, Diana Yeates, James Yeates' family and the police. One by one, consultant doctors from major Sydney hospitals were interrogated with few contributing much of value.

There was extensive evidence from neighbours around the Yeates property who had detected his car in the driveway with its door open, lights on and engine running for some hours before they, in desperation, alerted Mrs Yeates to the fact. The neighbours also described another motor vehicle which had called in at the Yeates' house on a number of occasions. Although some believed that Hedberg's widow had died from heart disease, there was a strong suggestion by others that she had been poisoned by Hedberg's injections.

The Coroner became increasingly impatient with the intense legal wrangling about his role and his allowing the admission of much evidence which appeared not to lead anywhere when there were many more witnesses waiting to give evidence. Relationships between all legal parties continued to deteriorate. Much was made of the fact that Hedberg had returned to work soon after his first wife's hasty cremation and had coped well with her death.

After the Christmas-New Year break, the inquest recommenced on January 17, 1961 when pathological and pharmacological opinions were again that Yeates' head injury had not occurred simply by a fall in the garage and that he had been injected with a very large dose of adrenaline, probably while still alive. Several doctors gave conflicting accounts of what they knew about the relationships between Hedberg and Yeates and between their families.

Nonetheless, Diana Yeates' senior counsel and her solicitor (an elder brother of past Australian prime minister, John Howard) insisted that the Coroner was confused about his role and was allowing inadmissible evidence which was damaging to Diana Yeates. Her counsel maintained that the press had been freely invited to examine photographs and other exhibits which should have been protected at that time.

It was publicised that James Yeates and Diana Yeates had not been sleeping in the same bedroom for at least six weeks. Coroner Rodgers warned Hedberg's senior counsel: *'There is a great deal of evidence to support a finding of murder or manslaughter.'* Shortly after, he added: *'There is not a single piece of evidence which, in itself or through interpretation, points to murder or manslaughter. So far as appears from the evidence, accident was the cause of injury.'* On and on the conflicting statements ran to confuse many who listened or watched.

Such was the confusion that Diana Yeates was advised by her barrister to refuse to answer the Coroner's questions. The Coroner responded: *'I do not feel justified in this case, if Mrs Yeates and Dr Hedberg do not wish to go into the witness box, to compel them to do so.'* Underlying all this distressing interplay, there was the issue of 'the other [possible] murder' — that of Hedberg's first wife.

There was a growing view amongst observers that Coroner Rodgers was not adequately investigating Yeates death for reasons which were not obvious with an agenda that nobody else understood. He finally summed up by saying that he regarded the whole case as being surrounded by mysterious features and much unfortunate publicity. He agreed that there was much evidence of a relationship between Hedberg and Diana Yeates although there were excessive problems of 'hearsay'.

He finished by saying: '*So far as this enquiry is concerned, there is not one scintilla of evidence which in any way involves Dr Hedberg or Mrs Yeates in the death of Dr Yeates. I find that Dr James Macrae Yeates was feloniously slain by a person or persons unknown.*'

Coroner Rodgers' inquest had also raised the issue of Hedberg's involvement, if any, in the death of his first wife five months earlier when there had been accusations that he had wanted to poison her. When Rodgers was unable to recommend a criminal trial on any count, the NSW Bar Association and other legal authorities complained bitterly about his conduct of the inquiry and that of the police, the media and the testimony of some witnesses.

After the trial's dust had settled, Hedberg told reporters that he felt better than he had for four months. Diana Yeates expressed her relief that it was all over. Later, she gave an interview in which she said: '*The rumours that began were unbelievable. As I expected, the Coroner didn't believe them. I would like to pay tribute to my legal advisers, Mr Gordon Samuels and Mr Stanley Howard. I am glad these vicious rumours have been put to rest. My only regret is the mystery of Jim's death is not yet cleared up.*'

Postscript

On the next day, the NSW 'Government Gazette' proclaimed that a new Act had come into force on February 1, 1961 whereby a Coroner could no longer help the police in an enquiry into a death or make a finding of murder or manslaughter and then commit a person to trial. The Bar Council and the NSW Bar Association claimed that Coroner Rodgers had let the inquest run twice as long as it should have and that Hedberg and Diana Yeates had been bullied. The media wondered if anybody had effectively interviewed Diana Yeates.

James Yeates' will bequeathed everything to Diana. Hedberg's practice suffered as a result of the publicity surrounding the inquest. Nobody came forward when an offer of £1,000 reward for information leading to the conviction of Yeates' killer was posted. Yeates' siblings sought a Royal Commission without success. The police said that their files would remain open although many court documents could not be found at that time.

Hedberg died in 2001 when he and Diana had been together for 37 years. It should be emphasised that he had never been referred to the NSW Medical Board or to any other disciplinary body concerning his possible relationship with Yeates, or with his first wife's death, or with any other form of misconduct.

Chapter 11

Brief notes on well-known British Cases

T he following cases have been selected more or less at random for features which set them apart from the nature of most Australian cases such as reported above. Again, salient features are freely available from public records though not in such detail as the Australian cases.

Seyi Awotona was a consultant obstetrician before she was sacked from a hospital in Newcastle, England for 'gross personal misconduct'. She had raised concerns about the standard of care at the hospital where she was employed in 1998. In 2007, an industrial tribunal found that she had been dismissed because she had been collecting evidence against her bosses for a racial discrimination claim. (It seems likely that she was regarded as a 'disruptive' doctor. See Chapters 9 and 10 here.) Six years later and eighteen months after the tribunal found that her sacking had been unfair, she wanted to return to work but the hospital refused to take her back. She turned to a tribunal to clarify the issue.

While she and the hospital attempted to reconcile their differences, hospital managers insisted that, after such a long period of interruption to her work, she required retraining. Other senior doctors at the hospital threatened to resign if she was reinstated. In 2005, by court order she was reinstated by The South Tyneside Health Care Trust and awarded one million pounds in compensation for wrongful interruption of her work and income.

Ashoka Prasad was a psychiatrist who was removed from medical registers in both Canada and Australia before he was also investigated by the General Medical Council in Britain in 1988. It seems that Commonwealth registration bodies did not then have formal mechanisms for sharing information about doctors who had been suspended from practice somewhere else.

In 1987, while in Melbourne working for the Victorian Mental Health Research Institute, Prasad was involved in an investigation into schizophrenia. An enquiry decided that Prasad had fabricated his data and he did not actually hold claimed degrees of PhD and DSc. The Victorian Medical Practitioners Board deregistered him.

When Prasad was working later in a university in Nova Scotia, a letter bearing a forged signature was sent to the British Medical Journal stating that Prasad had been exonerated of any Australian charges. Unfortunately for Prasad, the alleged author of the letter had died months before its date.

In 1990 Prasad's name was also removed from the register in British Colombia where he had falsely claimed to have been nominated for a Nobel Peace Prize. In 1994, forged documents arrived at the Victorian Medical Board from India accusing Prasad's senior colleagues in Australia of narcotics offences.

In 1997, Prasad was a locum consultant in England when professors at the Universities of Edinburgh and Birmingham received letters on an official South African medical letterhead in a handwritten envelope carrying a British postmark. The letter stated that the professor who had charge of Prasad's original research in Melbourne had been struck off the South African medical register for narcotics trafficking. The addressing on the envelope appeared to have been written by Prasad.

As far as is known, he has not been restored to any Commonwealth medical register.

Harold Shipman, a British GP, was accused of murdering middle aged or elderly women after forging their wills in which he was a significant beneficiary. He was tried for one murder in 1957 but acquitted. He then ran a solo general practice in Manchester until he was taken into custody for the murder of four other women. Police exhumed another body before charging Shipman with a further 28 murders involving the forging of wills with the intention of receiving £300,000. The police planned to scrutinise 3,000 prescriptions written by Shipman to obtain drugs with which to kill his patients.

John Adams, another British GP, worked in a genteel English seaside-resort where he persuaded a wealthy widow to write a will leaving him money. He then gave her a lethal dose of drugs. Gossip and hearsay soon reached such a peak that local police had little choice but to undertake detailed enquiries. When the media conducted their own 'trial', the evidence against Adams became overwhelming. One headline mentioned 400 patients whose wills were favourable to Adams.

Clifford Ayling was jailed for four years in 2000 after being convicted of 13 counts of indecent assault on his patients when a GP in Kent, England. Complaints had originally been made in the early 1980s but he was not investigated thoroughly. He continued practising for nearly 30 years before he was finally deemed by the GMC to be unfit to be registered. The National Health Service was later charged with seriously inadequate investigation of doctors accused of sexual misbehaviour.

Richard Neale was an obstetrician and gynaecologist who practised in England despite being struck off the register in Canada in 1985 after an investigation into the deaths of two patients. Regardless of that history, he had been allowed to return to work at hospitals in Yorkshire, Leicester and London before being removed from the UK Medical Register in 2000. He had been found guilty of 34 charges of incompetent medical care. The General Medical Council apologised for its mishandling of the matter and assured the National Health Service that the situation could not happen again.

David Southall was a British paediatrician who was investigated in February 2007 for wrongly accusing a father of infanticide. An examination of Southall's lengthy record as a 'witness for the prosecution' in cases of suspected infanticide ('cot-death') indicated that he might have been holding nearly 5,000 children's files which were not properly stored in hospital record systems.

Southall had become famous as a witness after he had watched a TV interview with a grieving father whom he then accused of killing his two babies. Although the mother was later convicted of the murders, her conviction was quashed when other evidence showed that the children had died naturally. In 2005, London's High Court ruled that Southall could stay on the medical register only under strict conditions.

The General Medical Council, however, chose to conduct its own hearing into Southall's conduct. It appeared that Southall might have given evidence in several criminal court proceedings which were not made aware of the existence and contents of his private records. A 10-year review of his files was to be undertaken.

Andrew Wakefield became prominent when he and others reported (*Lancet* 1998) dangers associated with a combined mumps, measles and rubella vaccine for children. His study included only a dozen subjects but created an international scare which resulted in 25 times more reports of measles in England and Wales between 1997 and 2008. According to the General Medical Council, Wakefield's 'research' involved financial rewards for studied children and a large personal reward from lawyers acting for parents who believed that their children had been damaged by triple immunisation.

Adam Cresswell's report of January 30, 2010 in *The Australian* indicated that Wakefield's conduct had been considered by the Council to be unqualified, unethical and callous. Acknowledged expert authorities found no significant evidence that the vaccine could be blamed for autism, gut problems or delayed neurological development. Wakefield's deregistration was considered imminent.

Epilogue

I have tried to understand how and why doctors may stray from where they always wanted to be and put their once blameless reputations at risk. It is difficult to know how and where they can practise if they are sidelined or banished from the only work they ever wanted to do. Who knows how it was that, throughout its long history, similar principles of desirable medical conduct were developed across the world despite little collaboration? The profusion of regulations suggests that default is always possible.

No doubt, religious teaching featured largely in the formulation of rules and penalties — creating the concept of needing to be 'registered' to practise such an esoteric, dangerous and distinguished occupation. For that, they must be considered fit to empathise with, touch, comfort and share the lonely agonies of others' distress. That role implies the unattainable expectation of 'total' integrity. That such a demand in some way exceeds the capabilities of doctors should come as no surprise. Sadly, the price paid for default may include the irretrievable loss of rare medical resources forged by time and high hopes.

I reiterate that my writing does not imply in any way that I have formed judgements on these doctors' intellect, principles, moral integrity or performance. My objective has been to present the predicaments in which they have found themselves during otherwise blameless professional lives.

Bibliography

AAP, *Edelsten tries to re-enter the ranks of doctors*, Fairfax Digital, 25 November 2003

ABC News, *McBride cleared to return to work*, Sydney, 09 November 1998

ABC News, Sydney, 04 November 2003

ABC News, *Edelsten appeals to NSW Medical Tribunal*, 24 November 2003

ABC News, *Australian doctor acquitted of murder in Uganda*, 12 December, 2006

ABC News, *British Police investigate hospital terrorist cell*, 03 July 2007

ABC News, *Second doctor detained in Brisbane terrorist raids (Mohamed Haneef)*, 03 July 2007

ABC News, *Don't pick on overseas doctors: Overseas Doctors' Association*, ABC, 03 July 2007

ABC News, *Medical Board to discipline chief over Patel affair*, Bundaberg, 20 November 2007

ABC News, *Retrial over Doctor's Killing*, News Ltd, 15 May 2008

ABC News, *Fed Govt 'never considered' Haneef innocent*, 1 July 2008

ABC News, *'Stillborn baby' comes back to life in hospital fridge*, 19 August 2008

ABC News, *Organs removed before Donors are 'Dead'*, 20 October 2008

ABC News, *Retrial convicts Gassy of mental health chief's murder*, 06 May 2009

ABC News, *Jury considers Gassy retrial verdict*, Sydney, 06 May 2009

ABC News, *Patel to face manslaughter trial in March*, 14 August 2009

Ackland, R, *How the Haneef affair became 'Carry on Coppers'*, *Sydney Morning Herald*, 23 August 2008

Addict doctor's 10-year ban, *Sydney Morning Herald*, 05 November 2003

Albrecht, H, Notes on conversation, dated April 29, 1998

Al-Ghazal, S, *Medical Ethics in Islamic History at a Glance*, London, JISHIM, 2004

Archives in Brief 72 — Records of the NSW Medical Board, 1986

Baker, R, McKenzie, N, *Kickback claims being taken 'very seriously'*, *The Age*, 13 March 2008

Baker, R, McKenzie, N, *Money trail in the US medical devices investigation leads to Melbourne*, *The Age*, 12 March 2008

Barnard, Christiaan, Personal communications and British Medical Journal, 22 December 2001

Blacket, R, Personal letter to author, 12 December 1987

Bowring, A, Affidavit to CEO, Prince of Wales Hospital, August 1986

Browning, M, *Chelmsford victim turns to UN*, London Guardian, 15 March 2000

Chandler, J, *Scandal of 'Dr Death'*, *The Age*, Bundaberg, 28 May 2005

Childs, W, Entry in *Your Australian Business Directory*, Sydney, 2008

Citizens' Commission on Human Rights, *Criminal Acts as Therapy*, 1969

Clift, E, *Rethinking Medical Ethics*, Boloji, 06 May 2008

Code of Professional Conduct, NSW Medical Board

Colburn, D, (Jayant Patel) Oregon-Live: March 11, 2008

Controversial doctor's court cases to be reviewed, London: Reuters, 20 February 2007

Collicott, P, *Errant Doctors*. American College of Surgeons, Chicago, 15 April 2008

Court of Criminal Appeal, South Australia, Gassy v The Queen (A2/2006), Judgement, 22 December 2005

Crow, S, *A Prescription for the Rogue Doctor,* University of New Orleans, 2003

Current Deregistered Doctors, NSW Medical Board internet listing, continuing

Deacon, G, *Letter concerning anaesthetic deaths, The Australian*, November 2007

DeBakey, ME, Multiple personal communications, 1973-2008

Define moment of death, says Pope, The Australian, 08 November 2008

Diamond, M, *Inside Madness: The Murder of a Psychiatrist*, September 2006

Disciplinary Action/Misconduct and Health Law News, Australian Legal Information, various years

Disciplinary Actions Taken, Bull Am Coll Surg, March 2008

District Court of NSW — *Medical Tribunal*, Sydney, CaseLawNSW, various years, ongoing

Douglas, F, Letter to author, 14 August 1986

Dyer, C, *Better systems needed to curb rogue doctors*, London: BMJ, 18 September 2004

Dyer, C, *British GP* (Shipman) *may face further murder charges,* London: BMJ, 17 October 1998

Edelsten, G, *Geoff Edelsten's history, career and academic accolades*, Copyright 2007, Prof. Geoffrey Edelsten and Licensors, 13 May 2008

Editorial: *Couch to the Bedroom, Sydney Morning Herald*, 17 December 2005

Editorial: *Islamic Culture and the Medical Arts,* US National Library of Medicine, Maryland, 15 April 1998

Editorial: *Medical error statistics,* Australian Legal Information, various dates 2007

Editorial: *Patients put down, The Daily Telegraph*, 12 September 2005

Editorial: *The patient must have faith in the systems*, *The Age*, 13 March 2008

Editorial: *Whipping the Doctors*, London, *The Spectator*, 17 June 2000

Executive, NSW Medical Board, *Reporting Statistics*, 09 May 2008

Faunce, K, *Hipbones and hip pockets*, *The Age*, 13 March 2008

Federation of State Medical Boards, Dallas, Texas, USA, 2001-2006

Flatley, C, *Patel didn't take advice from staff*, *Sydney Morning Herald*, 11 February, 2009

Forum: Medical Malpractice, Australia, 2007

Freedom of Information Application to Dept. of Justice and Attorney General

Gale, A, Letter to NSW Health Department

Galletly, C, *Crossing Professional Boundaries in Medicine: The slippery slope to patient sexual exploitation*, MJA, 2004.

Gassy v The Queen, Appeal, 22 December 2005

Geason, S, *Dark trance — Dr Harry Bailey and the Chelmsford Private Hospital scandal*, July 2007

Gerathy, J, *Response to JSW letter regarding 'sham' enquiry in 1986 and Crawford's role*, 18 June 2008

Haire, N, *Hymen or the Future of Marriage*, London, *International Journal of Psychoanalysis*, 1927, *Becoming a Sexologist*: Norman Haire, 2001

Hahn, J, Letter to CEO, Prince of Wales Hospital, 22 August, 1986

Hatton, J, *Dr William McBride Case*, NSW Parliament: Sydney, 01 December 1994

Health Care Complaints Commission (HCCC) — *Statement of Activities*, Sydney, 2007 and letter re '*care or treatment*' of patients, 31 August 2010

Incident Management in the NSW Public Health System, NSW Health CEC, January/June 2007

Judgement: Equity Division, Supreme Court NSW, No. 1213, 1987 — 04 September, 1987

Judgement: Supreme Court NSW Court of Appeal, Bannister v Walton, Sydney 30 April 1992

Kaplan, R, *Time for a new social contract between doctor and patient, Sydney Morning Herald,* 29 February 2008

Keim, T, *Questions about Patel's investigator put on hold, Courier Mail,* Brisbane, 29 July 2008

Kellett, C, *Media circus greets Patel, Sydney Morning Herald,* 09 February, 2009

Kennedy, J, *Problematic doctor behaviour, Three case studies,* School of Philosophy, U Syd, 2006

Kennedy, L, *Arrested doctor 'went on a road trip', Sydney Morning Herald,* 12 November 2002

Keren, D, *Medical experiments; teacher's guide to the holocaust,* Shamash: The Jewish Internet Consortium, Various letters, 2005

King, C, *Medical Ethics,* Univ. Pennsylvania, Encarta Online Encyclopaedia, 2007

Knightley, P, *Rogue doctors,* Personal communication with J Wright, 2006

Knightley, P, *The doctor is out,* Independent Monthly, Sydney, June 1990

Lamont, L, *Repentant Edelsten wants to practise again,* UNSW Law, Fairfax Digital, 25 November 2003

Labour Force: Medical, Australian Government Health & Welfare, Canberra, 2007

Lee, T, *Medical Ethics in Ancient China,* Bull, Hist Med, 1943

Leigh, B, Report on Committee of Enquiry, November, 1986

Leigh, B, Letters of August 27, 1986 and undated

Limprecht, E, *Dr Andrew Hollo ... cleared of trying to murder one of his patients,* Simply 4 Doctors: 17 November 2004

Lindeberg, K, *Haneef witnesses risk civil law suits, The Australian,* 09 May 2008

Lindeberg, K, *Note on Heiner affair*, Brisbane, 27 April 2008

Loong, E, Letter to NSW Health Department, 06 April 2000

Lusetich, R, *Patel close to being granted bail*, Editorial: Ministerial media statements, 26 April 2005

Man comes back to life as doctors prepare to remove his organs, *Sydney Morning Herald*, 11 June 2008

McBride, W, *Birth defects in children of patients who were prescribed thalidomide*, London: The Lancet, December 1961

McEwin, R, Personal letters to author

McKensey, P, Letter to Independent Monthly, August 1990

McNeill, P, *Medical serial killers*, ABC Health Report, 18 July 2005

McNeill, P, *Nuremberg Trials*, A Companion in Bioethics: Blackwell, 1998

Martin, B, '*Suppression of dissent*' *documents* and M Crawford's response to charge of misrepresentation, University of Wollongong, May 1997 and 1998

Media Release: *Premier Carr announces new $55 million Clinical Excellence Commission*, NSW Department of Health, 08 April 2004

Mee, R, Personal letters to author

Mayo Clinic, Rochester, Minnesota, report: *Matthew Crawford's fellowship*, direct communication, 1986

Medical Disciplinary Tribunal, Judgement re Geoffrey Lancelot Davis, NSW Medical Board, undated

Medical Tribunal of NSW, *Re Jean Eric Gassy*, 01 August 1997

Miller, G, Letter to author, 23 February 2009

Murnaghan, G, Letter to author, 02 July, 1980

Nainggolan, L, *Cardiologists sued over UMDNJ Kickback Scheme*, Medscape, 2008

NSW Medical Board, *New Cosmetic Surgery Guidelines*, July 2008

NSW Medical Board, *A decision of the Medical Tribunal of NSW in relation to Dr William McBride and the Medical Practices Act*, Sydney, 29 April 1996

NSW Medical Board, *Annual Reports and Tribunal Findings*, 1986-2007

NSW Parliament, *Death of Mrs Shirley Byrne*, Sydney, 02 May 2006

O Death, when is thy sting? London: *Economist*, 02 October 2008

Pope slams human organ trade, warns on transplants, Medscape (Reuters Health Information), 2008

Program in Human Rights and in Medicine, University of Minnesota, 09 February 2006

Queensland Public Hospitals, *Commission of Enquiry*, Bundaberg, 2008

Reports of surgeons and anaesthetists on Prince of Wales Hospital Operating Rooms, November, 1995

Research@National Heart Foundation, Grant recipients, *(Mr Gerrit Reimers)*, October 2007

Saunders, C, *What are the risks — both legal and personal — involved in peer review of colleagues?* Simply 4 Doctors, 20 January 2005

Savage, M, *Sacked doctor's fight continues*, BBC News, London, 29 September 2004

Smyth, T, Response to letter re 'sham' enquiry, Prince of Wales Hospital, 1986

Smyth, T, Multiple letters to supportive parents, Prince of Wales Hospital, 1986

Solomon, M, *Editorial: Healthcare professionals and dual loyalty*, Medscape General Medicine, 2005

South Korean cloning scientist looking overseas: report, Seoul: Reuters, 11 June 2007

Stephens, A, *Where the dead men lie*, Angus & Robertson, Sydney: 1897

Sutton, C, *The needle in the heart murder, and the mysterious death of Dr Yeates*, Sydney: Allen & Unwin, 2003 and more than 600 Sydney media articles

Swan, N, *Investigating Scientific Fraud*, ABC Health Report, 17 August 1998

Swan, N, *Psychiatrist is investigated by GMC,* London: BMJ, 12 September 1998

Sweeney, C, *UMP backs defence of disgraced anaesthetist*, United Medical Protection, 12 November 2003

Sweet, M, *Inside Madness: The Murder of a Psychiatrist* and *Murder in Medicine*, Sydney, 1986

Tabakoff, N, *Life and loves of man bucking his past*, Geoffrey Edelsten on jail, Brynne Gordon, *The Daily Telegraph*, 26 September 2009

The text of the Covenant laid down by Hippocrates, University of Minnesota, 2006–2007

Thomas, H, *Rogue agencies profiting over doctor shortage*, Press Clippings, Parliament of Australia, 30 April 2007

Wallace, N, *Hospitals blamed for series of deaths, Sydney Morning Herald*, 26 August 2008

Watson, R, Letter to Independent Monthly, July 1990

Weakness of Mohamed Haneef case exposed, News Ltd, 16 May 2008

Werth, G, Waller, E, *The role of the expert witness*, Bull Am Coll Surg, December 2005

Wikipedia: various entries, *Jayant Patel.*

Wikipedia: various entries, *Medical Ethics.*

Wikipedia: *Saints Cosmas & Damian.*

Wooldridge, M, 'Beattie must not shift blame to others', *The Australian*, 07 July 2010

Woolridge, J, Letter to NSW Health Department, 06 April, 2000

Wright, J, 'CV invented', In, *Suppression of Dissent*, Brian Martin, UOW, 1998

Wright, J, *Notes, diaries, interviews, hospital politics*, Recorded in 'Suppression of Dissent' documents, A/Professor B Martin, 1988

Yabsley, M, *Medical Tribunal Enquiry into Dr McBride*, NSW Parliament, 26 November 1992